Lymphedema

Lawrence L. Tretbar · Cheryl L. Morgan · B.B. Lee ·
Simon J. Simonian · Benoit Blondeau

Lymphedema

Diagnosis and Treatment

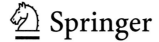 Springer

Lawrence L. Tretbar, MD, ScD, FACS, FRSM (Eng)
Clinical Associate Professor of Surgery
University of Kansas School of Medicine
Kansas City, KS
USA

Cheryl L. Morgan, PhD
Adjunct Faculty
Rockhurst University
Kansas City, MO
USA

Byung-Boong Lee, MD, PhD, FACS
Professor of Surgery
Georgetown University School of Medicine
Washington, DC
USA

Simon J. Simonian, MD, ScM, ScD, FACS
Clinical Professor of Surgery
Georgetown University School of Medicine
Washington, DC
USA

Benoit Blondeau, MD
Assistant Professor of Surgery
University of Missouri-Kansas City
School of Medicine
Kansas City, MO
USA

British Library Cataloguing in Publication Data
Lymphedema : diagnosis and treatment
  1. Lymphedema
  I. Tretbar, Lawrence L., 1933–
  616.4'2
  ISBN-13: 9781846285486

Library of Congress Control Number: 2007930548

ISBN: 978-1-84628-548-6   e-ISBN: 978-1-84628-739-0

9 8 7 6 5 4 3 2 1

springer.com

Foreword

Lower extremities do not only allow the upper part of the body containing heart, lungs, and alimentary tract to be transferred from one place to another, but they also carry our brain where it commands. We live longer, our brains work longer, our legs become worn out. Mentally fully capable older individuals become home-, chair-, bed-confined. Sick legs eliminate them from professional and social life. Any new information on diagnosis and treatment of diseases of lower extremities is desperately needed—not only for education of medical professionals but also for patients, who are often the earliest "diagnosers" of this illness. One of the pathological conditions affecting human legs is edema. Of course, edema is only a symptom of an ongoing process in soft and hard tissues of the limb. Hundreds of millions of people around the world either already suffer from pathological events in their extremities or will suffer in the future. Each pathological process in the limbs involves the lymphatic system. The lymph system is a regulatory and defence organization regulating water and chemical environment of cells, participates in healing and defends against penetrating microorganisms. There are pathological factors specifically damaging the limb lymphatic system, but this system may also be adversely affected by diseases specific for other tissues (e.g. vein, tendons, ligaments, bones and nerves). The book *Lymphedema* by Lawrence L. Tretbar, Cheryl L. Morgan, B.B. Lee, Simon J. Simonian, and Benoit Blondeau gives a comprehensible insight into all aspects of the lymphatic system under physiological and pathological conditions. The authors are authorities in the field of lymphology and phlebology and managed to present their knowledge in a most condensed fashion. The book has been written in simple language and can be useful even for those who are far away from clinical medicine. Multiple color figures do not only perfectly illustrate what happens to the extremity in case of damage of the lymphatics and lymph nodes, they are so expressive that having seen them no professional or patient would neglect early limb swelling and postpone referring to or seeing a specialist.

Waldemar L. Olszewski
Professor of Surgery
Former President, International Society of Lymphology

Preface

Lymphology is finally recognized by American medicine as a distinct medical specialty. Its acceptance has no doubt been hastened by a more complete understanding of the embryologic and microscopic changes found in lymphatic diseases. Technologic advances (e.g., scanning electron microscopy or lymphangioscintigraphy) have also contributed to our understanding of the lymphatic system.

As an increasing amount of knowledge emerges from the study of the lymphatics, it is clearly apparent that the venous system is intimately associated with it. This fact is readily observed by the authors.

Members of the public, as well as health professionals, are looking for new and reliable information on lymphedema. As cancer survivors age, their risk of developing lymphedema increases. Unfortunately, one common source of information, the Internet, may present information that is incomplete, misleading, inadequate, and often inappropriate.

Using evidence-based sources and their own extensive clinical experience, our authors have assembled an impressive amount of clinical and research material. They have created a pool of information that should help us form a more unified concept of the lymphatic system, and its many aberrations.

One goal of this book is to provide some simple guidelines for the physician who must direct and follow the patient's progress during treatment of lymphatic or venous disorders. This requires a basic understanding of the vascular disorders, available interventions and the need for life-long follow-up.

Another goal is to inform a knowledgeable public that lymphedema is a problem that can be treated—successfully. No longer should a person accept the concept that lymphedema is something they "must learn to live with."

It is our collective experience that patients who face this complex, potentially disfiguring and disabling medical problem achieve superior outcomes when managed by a knowledgeable physician and an experienced therapist. They also demonstrate greater adherence to the recovery program.

Lastly, only through the concerted efforts of the "team," physicians, therapists, and patients, can the insurance carriers be convinced that people with lymphatic diseases deserve the same economic support as those with other vascular diseases.

My gratitude to the authors, especially Dr. Cheryl L. Morgan, for their contributions, and to Emily Iker, MD, for the use of her many photographs.

Lawrence L. Tretbar

Contents

Foreword *by Waldemar L. Olszewski* v

Preface vii

1 Structure and Function of the Lymphatic System 1
   Lawrence L. Tretbar

2 Differential Diagnosis of Lymphedema 12
   Simon J. Simonian, Cheryl L. Morgan, Lawrence L. Tretbar,
   and Benoit Blondeau

3 Classification and Staging of Lymphedema 21
   Cheryl L. Morgan and B.B. Lee

4 Lymphatic Malformation 31
   B.B. Lee

5 Medical Management of Lymphedema 43
   Cheryl L. Morgan

6 Surgical Management of Lymphedema 55
   B.B. Lee

7 Chronic Lymphovenous Disease 64
   Lawrence L. Tretbar

Index 71

1

Structure and Function of the Lymphatic System

Lawrence L. Tretbar

Early Investigations

Like many anatomical discoveries, the early anatomists described the lymphatic system in morphologic terms. Little was recognized about the function of the system until some centuries later.

The visibility of the blood circulatory system made it an easy system to study and encouraged early investigators to examine it thoroughly. Nevertheless, many curious anatomists recognized the differences between the blood circulatory system and the lymphatic system.

Hippocrates described "chyle" in the intestinal tract. Of interest, too, is his equation of lymphatic states with emotional states. He described 3 lymphatic temperaments: phlegm (lymph and chyle), yellow bile, and black bile (1,2).

Similarly, during the Middle Ages "physiks," i.e. academic physicians, promulgated the concept of 4 "humors" within the body: blood, black bile, yellow bile, and phlegm. According to this belief, if you had too much phlegm you became phlegmatic, too much black bile caused melancholy, and an excess of yellow bile made you to feel bilious. An overflow of blood allowed you to become sanguine, clever, and thoughtful. We still talk about humors, for example one may be in a good or bad humor. We still describe pulmonary mucous as phlegm. While the descriptive terms phlegmatic, sanguine, bilious, and melancholy are perhaps archaic, they nevertheless remain a part of our language.

During the early 17th century, Aselli pointed out the differences between lymph vessels and veins and was the first to describe the lacteals, "venae albae et lacteae," or white and milklike veins (3,4). He died before publishing his findings, but fortunately 2 colleagues proceeded to publish them in 1627, a year after his death (5) (Figure 1-1).

A young Swedish anatomist, Rudbeck, further identified the nature of the lymphatic system. He recognized it as a distinct system, separate from the blood circulatory system, that ultimately drains its contents into the upper veins (6,7).

During this period of discovery, Harvey, a former student of Fabricius in Padua, defined the blood circulatory system. However, his major publication in 1628, a year after Aselli's, made no mention of the lymphatics and only described the circulation of blood through its various compartments (8,9). Later, he did make many comments on the findings of other anatomists regarding their contributions to lymphatic research.

The English school of investigation provided other contributions to the understanding of the lymphatics. The Hunter brothers in London established the Anatomy School on Windmill Street (10) (Figure 1-2).

Mascagni, a professor of anatomy in Siena, created and published a magnificent compendium of work in 1787. It contributed enormously to the understanding of the lymphatic system, especially its anatomy. Its illustrations are as useful today as they were then (11) (Figure 1-3).

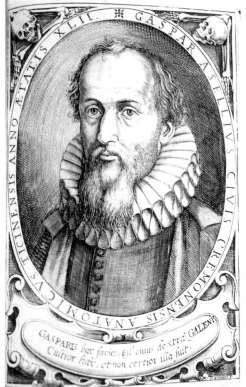

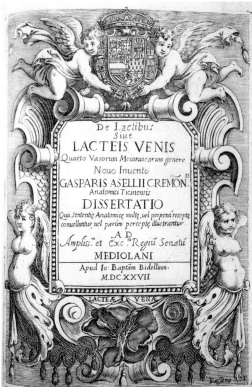

A

B

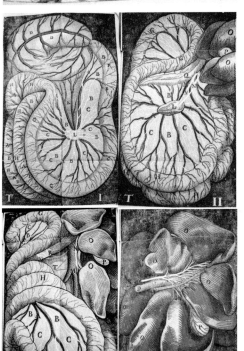

C

FIGURE 1-1. (A) Gaspar Aselli (1581–1626), age 42 years. (B) The frontispiece of Aselli's posthumously published dissertation shows the expected array of cherubs and armless angels. Note the image below the inscription; it is the same as T IIII shown in (C), but rotated counterclockwise and flopped left to right. This beautifully illustrated manuscript reveals in vivid detail the many contributions of the lymphatics to the body's circulation—the many intestinal lacteals and their joining lymphatic vessels. They were drawn from canine dissections, as attested by the multiple lobes of the liver. Peyer patches had not yet been described. (C) The first 3 plates show the intestine and its mesenteries. The final illustration shows the relationship of the lymph channels with the liver; its lobes and gall bladder are well depicted. These are probably the first anatomic illustrations to be published in color. These reproductions are from the original polychrome woodcuts, the portrait from a copperplate etching. Fold lines are evident from hundreds of years of use. (Image courtesy the Clendening History of Medicine Library, University of Kansas Medical Center.)

FIGURE 1-2. (A) William Hunter wrote that the lymphatic system created a "grand system for absorption, in men and quadrupeds." He combined the lacteals and lymphatics under the term "absorbent vessels," a common belief at the time. (B) John Hunter was probably more interested in "osteology" than circulation, but he had many thoughts about his and other's investigations. This classic etching reveals him as a thoughtful author. Of interest is the image of the skeleton of the famed Irish giant James Byrne, in the upper right. The skeleton is still on display in the Royal College of Surgeons' museum in London. (Photos courtesy the Royal Society of Medicine, London.)

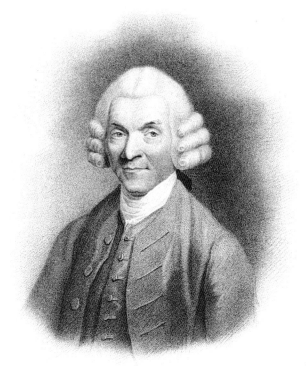

A

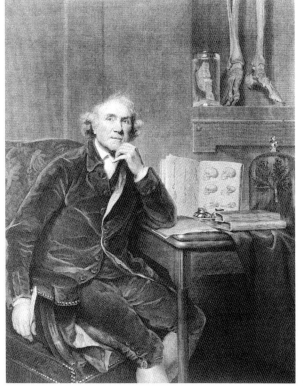

B

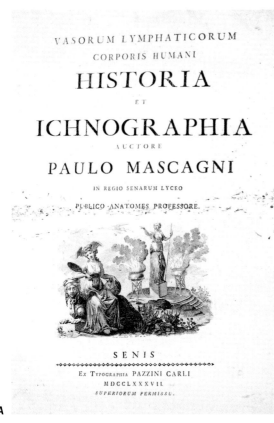

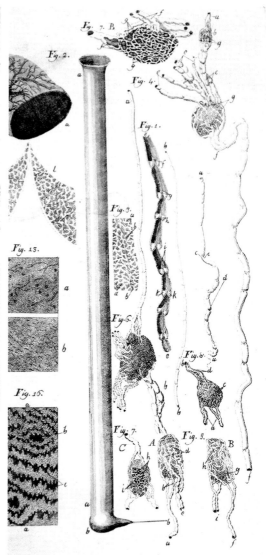

FIGURE 1-3. Paulo Mascagni (1755–1815) published this magnificent group of illustrations, a result of his meticulous dissections. (A) The frontispiece is of a classical nature and less ornate than earlier forms. (B) This illustration demonstrates the spectrum of lymphatic structures—peripheral lymphatics joining lymph nodes, intestinal lymphatics, and multiple valves within the vessels. The cylindrical structure is a pipette used to intubate and opacify lymph channels. (Image courtesy the Clendening History of Medicine Library, University of Kansas Medical Center.)

Lymphatic Embryology

The embryonic development of lymphatics was studied extensively during the beginning of the last century. Since then, however, this field of exploration has advanced slowly because of the lack of specific lymphatic markers, and because the issue of histogenetic origin remains controversial.

In the early 1900s, Sabin introduced a now widely accepted theory of lymphatic development. Her experimental evidence suggested that lymphangiogenesis parallels that of the venous system. She proposed that isolated primitive lymph sacs bud from endothelial cells during the sixth to seventh week of gestation and appear in the neck as extensions of the anterior cardinal veins (12). These primordial lymph sacs coalesce to form a large jugulo-axillary sac that eventually becomes the thoracic duct. Continued proliferation and segregation of distal lymphatic structures begins about the 10th week of gestation. Functional lymph nodes first appear in the axillae and in the primitive thymus and spleen at about the sixth week. Valves in superficial and deep lymphatics are seen during the fifth month.

Configuration of the Lymphatic System

The term microcirculation generally refers to the distal-most portion of the circulatory system, arterioles, capillaries, and venules. Capillaries are composed of a single layer of endothelial cells, many of which are separated by a cleft or pore. Precapillary sphincters, formed by a thin layer of muscle, help regulate the flow of blood into the capillary bed and the egress of fluids from them (11,13). Capillaries are the site of fluid, nutrient, and waste exchange.

Unlike blood vessels, the peripheral lymphatics are dead-ended. They originate in the distal-most tissues of the skin, muscles, visceral organs, lung, and intestine. Most lie within the neurovascular bundle that contains nerve elements, arteries, veins, and lymphatics. Therefore, lymph flow is centripetal, i.e. from distal to proximal (11,13–15) (Figure 1-4).

The lymphatic transport system is generally divided into 3 categories:

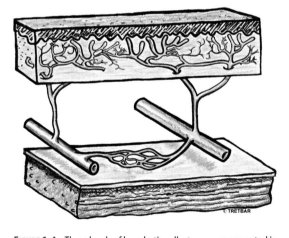

FIGURE 1-4. Three levels of lymphatic collectors are represented in this drawing. The upper layer is the skin with the originating, dead-ended collectors. In a normal situation, they are almost empty as they transport lymph. Subcutaneous tissue lies beneath the skin, and its own collecting systems carry the fluid to the fascia and muscles below. (Illustration by LL Tretbar.)

- the superficial system that drains the skin and subcutaneous tissues
- the deeper subfascial system that drains muscles, joints, synovial sheaths, and bones
- the visceral system that drains the small intestine, spleen, liver, thymus, and lungs

Lymphatic vessels are not normally present in avascular structures such as the epidermis, hair, nails, cartilage, and cornea, or in some vascularized organs like the brain and retina (13,15–19).

From their distal origins, the lymphatics continue as 2 distinct structures: transport vessels and solid organs. Collecting vessels transport lymphatic fluid to lymph nodes and ultimately to the neck veins (15,16,19,20).

Prelymphatic Tissue Channels

Prelymphatic channels are the original part of the lymph-collecting system. Although these tiny vascular structures contain no endothelium and are not usually considered lymphatic channels, they direct interstitial fluid to the capillaries (16,17).

Lymph Capillaries

Capillaries are valveless and lined with a single-cell layer of continuously overlapping endothelial cells. Reticulated, filamentous, fibrous strands anchor the capillary to the surrounding tissue fibrils. They play an important role in regulating fluid flow into and out of the capillary by alternatively stretching and relaxing (13,14,18). This structure makes the capillary quite permeable; it permits the absorption and drainage of enormous quantities of protein-rich lymph from the extracellular spaces. Lymphatic capillaries have been improperly called terminal lymphatics; they originate in the periphery, rather than terminating there (18,19,21).

Lymph Precollectors

Sometimes considered the initial lymph vessel, the precollectors contain 1 or more layers of muscle cells. They are singly or doubly valved (bicuspid), may contain collagenous fibers, and are dispersed from 6 to 20 cm apart. Their main function is to initiate flow through the chain of lymphatic structures, whereas valves maintain centripetal flow (14,17,19).

Lymph Collectors

At this level, collectors represent the main transport mechanism for lymph and begin to resemble other vascular structures. Their walls are composed of an endothelial-lined intima, a media composed of muscle cells and collagen fibers and an adventitia of collagen fibers that extend into the perivascular tissues. Vasa vasora, the tiny blood vessels that nourish the lymphatic tissues, begin to emerge (15,19,20).

The lymph vessel lying between valves is called a lymphangion. Liberally supplied with sympathetic and parasympathetic nerves, lymphangions form a unique muscular unit that initiates spontaneous contractions (20–26) (Figure 1-5).

Peyer Patches

Another unique situation occurs within the small intestine. In the submucosa of the distal ileum, the lining is a velvety surface of villi—millions of fingerlike projections that increase the total surface area. Peyer patches form the lymphatic interface of the mucosa with the products of digestion. After the digestion of fat, these substances in the form of chylomicrons, e.g. free fatty acids,

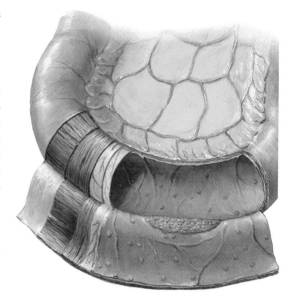

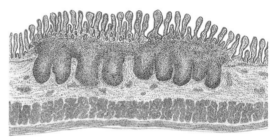

FIGURE 1-6. Peyer patches are easily seen within the small intestine in this illustration. A unique component of the lymphatic system, they provide another method for the body to absorb fats. (Netter medical illustrations, used with permission of Elsevier. All rights reserved.)

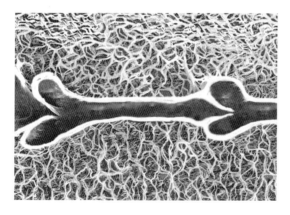

FIGURE 1-5. A lymphangion is seen between 2 valves. Lymphatic valves are similar to venous valves in their construction and function. Unlike venous structures, the lymphangion creates spontaneous contractions that propel the lymph toward the next valve or lymph node. (Modified and redrawn from Casteviholz A., *Lymphology* 31(3):101–118, computer enhanced to improve visual clarity.)

cholesterol, phospholipids, and lipoproteins, are absorbed into the lymphatics, where the fluid is called chyle (20,21,26). The lymphatic vessels conducting lymph from the intestinal mucosa to the mesenteric nodes are known as lacteals, a term which suggests milk; in an early observation in a well-fed dog, the vessels appeared milky, thus the term lacteal (20). Any surgeon who has had to operate on an accident victim in the middle of the night recognizes the milky lacteals, opacified by late-evening snacks of fast foods (Figure 1-6).

Lymph Ducts

The ducts are the largest of the transport structures and mimic other vascular structures in their complexity. As these structures progress proximally, the space between valves increases, the tunica media thickens, and nerve endings increase (19,20,26).

As described above, lymph flow begins in tiny peripheral vessels and then proceeds to the nearest lymph node. From the medial foot and leg, the superficial lymphatics travel up the long saphenous vein to nodes in the popliteal space and the larger superficial nodal groups in the inguinal area. Lateral foot and leg lymph proceeds to the popliteal nodes (19,20,25,26).

Deeper lymphatics follow the blood vessels to end in the deep popliteal nodes. Of clinical interest are the lymph vessels that bypass the inguinal nodes and follow the sciatic nerve to the deep iliac nodes. These alternate routes permit lymph to be redirected when one system is nonoperative (15,20,22).

From the pelvic and lumbar nodal system, lymph is carried to the cisterna chyli, a large collecting basin situated in front of the first or second lumbar vertebra. It is the confluence of the many lymph channels from the lower extremities and continues cephalad as the large thoracic duct, the final pathway for transport of lymph into the neck veins. The intercostals and many other intervening lymph channels join the thoracic duct along the way (20,22,26) (Figure 1-7).

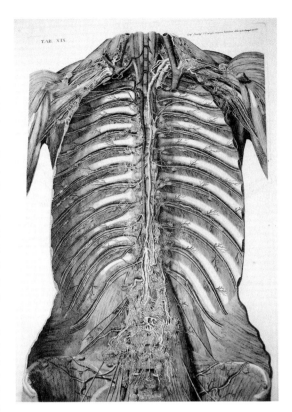

FIGURE 1-7. Mascagni provides another view of the lymphatics' pathways. This beautiful and anatomically correct illustration includes the pelvic distribution of multiple channels, nodes, the cisterna chyli, and the thoracic duct with its intercostal channels emptying into the subclavian veins. (Courtesy the Clendening History of Medicine Library, University of Kansas Medical Center.)

Lymph Nodes

Most people are familiar with lymph nodes because they become palpable when inflamed. Structurally, the node is kidney shaped and encompassed by a fibrous capsule containing collagen and single smooth muscle fibers. Many afferent lymph vessels enter the convex surface. Internally, trabeculae surround lymph sinuses where afferent collectors direct the influx of lymph to different parts of the sinuses, i.e. marginal, intermediate, and terminal. The concave surface is the hilum, where 1 and occasionally 2 efferent lymph channels direct lymph to the next set of nodes. Arterioles and venules enter and exit the node only at the hilum, as do tiny nerve fibers (19,21,23,26).

Lymph nodes are arranged in chains or groups and number as many as 600 to 700, most found in the abdominal and neck areas (13,26).

Wastes filtered by the nodes may consist of unwanted substances like high molecular proteins, fats, cellular debris, foreign organisms, viruses, and bacteria.

Large concentrations of macrophages, plasma cells, and lymphocytes within the nodal system initiate an immune response that kills live microbes and destroys other noxious substances. Lymph nodes produce lymphocytes and encourage their maturation along with reticuloendothelial cells, for example monocytes. Some lymphocytes remain in the node, whereas those passing through the node increase with the addition of those formed in the node and those contributed by the arterial and venous flow through the node (19,21,23,26).

Lymph is concentrated in the node, where almost half of its volume is removed by venous

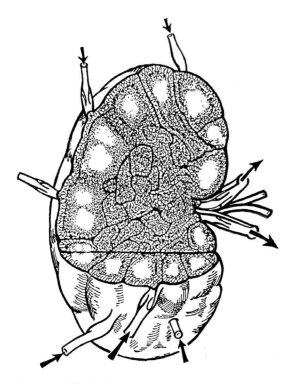

FIGURE 1-8. This familiar view of a lymph node shows the many afferent lymph vessels entering the node. Generally, there is 1efferent channel leaving the node, but there may be more. Arterioles and venules enter and exit only at the hilum. (Illustration modified from Schaeffer JP, ed, *Morris' Human Anatomy*, 11th ed. New York: Blakiston Company; 1953.)

flow. Slight pressure on the lymphatics, such as manual lymph drainage, further stimulates flow and therefore the production of lymphocytes (23) (Figure 1-8).

Functions of the Lymphatic System

Two or three major functions are attributed to the lymphatic system: the transport of lymph from the periphery of the body to the large veins of the neck; the maintenance of homeostasis, i.e. the balance of fluid volumes, pH, and electrolytes; and the regulation of immunity (22,26).

Interstitial Fluid/Edema

Lymph formation begins in the interstitial (intercellular) space, the space between somatic

cells. Fluid leaks from blood capillaries, filling the interstitial space. Most of the fluid is reabsorbed into the venules or the initial lymphatics (16,24).

Interstitial fluid is usually colorless and often considered serum, that is, blood without red blood cells and platelets. Its contents vary with different conditions, but in general it contains about 96% water plus these other items, proteins, lipids, carbohydrates, enzymes, glucose, urea, hormones, dissolved gases (carbon dioxide, oxygen), cells (lymphocytes, macrophages), unwanted toxins, bacteria and viruses, cellular debris, and other bodily wastes. Colloids are present as well—sodium, potassium, chloride, calcium, phosphorous, magnesium, and zinc or copper—in about the same concentrations as in plasma. When interstitial fluid finally enters an initial lymph capillary, it becomes lymph (16,21,23,24).

Edema is a condition in which the amount of interstitial fluid increases and the area becomes swollen with excess fluid. Factors that increase fluid discharge from the arteriovenous capillaries, such as trauma or infection, or that decreases its reabsorption into the lymphatics can cause edema (23,24).

Fluid Exchanges

According to Starling hypothesis, transport of fluids or particles through capillary filters depends on 4 variables: capillary blood pressure, interstitial tissue pressure, intravascular colloidal osmotic pressure (capillary), and extravascular colloidal osmotic pressure (tissue). It is important to understand the basic concepts of fluid and solute exchange between the arteriovenous circulation and the lymphatic system (18,25).

Diffusion

Many gases and solutes (dissolved solids) cross the arterial-capillary wall by diffusion, either through the endothelial cell wall or through structural clefts and pores. Diffusion is a passive process in which molecules move from an area of greater concentration to an area of lesser concentration. The type of diffusion usually depends on whether the gas or solute is lipid-soluble. Gases like O_2 or CO_2 are highly fat soluble and diffuse easily through the endothelial cell wall (18,23,24). Water-soluble substances, such as water, glucose, amino acids, and ionized substances, are not fat-soluble and must therefore pass through the intercellular clefts.

The process of diffusion is effective and efficient over short distances but less so at greater distances. When edema is present, the distance between cells increases and the transfer of nutrients and gases becomes more difficult (18,23).

Osmosis

Although diffusion accounts for much of the body's fluid exchange, osmosis remains the most important method of fluid transfer. Osmosis is the movement of fluid across a semipermeable membrane (the cell wall). A semipermeable membrane allows the passage of some molecules through it but not others. The movement of water is due to a difference in solute concentration, from an area of higher water concentration (less solute) to one of lower water concentration. The process is similar to diffusion, except that it is water and a few small molecules which pass through the membrane, rather than the opposite (19).

Two principal forces, hydrostatic pressure and osmotic pressure, regulate osmosis. Hydrostatic pressure is an external force transmitted to the blood vascular capillaries and the lymphatic capillaries. Arterial blood pressure, intrinsic lymphatic pressure, and gravity are the major hydrostatic forces applied to the 2 systems. Hydrostatic pressure in the initial lymphatics is negative, usually −5 to −6 cm water, and +6 cm in the kidney (23,24,26).

Osmotic pressure is determined by the type and amount of solute, especially protein, present in the fluid. The term osmotic pressure is misleading, because the "pressure" is actually a force attracting fluid through the membrane to the area of greater concentration; the greater the solute concentration, the greater the osmotic pressure. Osmotic pressure is also known as oncotic pressure (15,21,23).

In the physiologic state, it is estimated that between 2 to 4 L of interstitial fluid are filtered each day and returned via the lymphatics to the neck veins (23).

Lymph transport away from the interstitial space depends on a number of factors: local lymphatic contractions, contractions of adjacent muscles, arterial pulsations, changes in intraabdominal and thoracic pressures, and mechanical stimulation (16,23,25).

Spontaneous Contractions

Unlike the blood vascular system, in which the heart provides most of the propulsive force for circulation, the lymph system has its own distinct mode of propulsion. Lymph fluid is propelled by spontaneous segmental contractions within the lymphangion, the lymph channel between valves. The number of contractions within the lymphangion average about 6 to 15 per minute. Spontaneous contractions of the lymphangion can be augmented by external pressure, arterial pulsations, exercise, muscular contractions, and inspiration, among multiple other factors. As lymph enters the subclavian vein, where flow is rapid, a siphoning effect may also contribute to lymph movement (25,26).

Immune System

Every day the body is bombarded by thousands of foreign substances that try to gain entrance. The three major portals of entry into the body are the skin, the intestinal tract, and the lungs. Other internal products may appear as foreign substances to the body as well, for example cancer cells. Foreign materials become antigens, usually proteins, which incite an immune response that protects the body from these foreign invaders (23,27).

Natural, Nonspecific Immunity

Macrophages are mature monocytes and make up 5% to 10% of lymph. If there is infection or inflammation, other cellular elements may appear, including mast cells, eosinophils, granulocytes, platelets, and occasionally red blood cells.

Macrophages and monocytes are part of the mononuclear phagocyte system, once known as the reticuloendothelial system. They destroy many foreign substances by phagocytosis (literally, eating cells) and by secreting enzymes destructive to the antigen. They maintain a portion of the nonspecific immune system, the system that does not adapt to different antigens (17,27,29).

Specific Immunity

Many other cellular products make up lymph. Lymphocytes are the most abundant cell, representing about 80% to 85%, whereas they encompass only 20% to 40% of the blood's white cells. Found in both blood and lymph, they contribute to immune and phagocytic activities. Two types of lymphocytes develop: B cells that mature in the bone marrow, and T cells that mature in the thymus.

B cells are present in the germinal centers of lymph nodes and are found frequently in bone marrow and the spleen. When an antigen enters the body, B cells produce noncellular antibodies, or immunoglobulins, which contribute to the immune defense. Both cellular and noncellular substances complement the primary natural immune system (17,23,28).

When activated by a foreign substance, B cells may divide into 2 other types of cells: plasma cells and memory cells. Plasma cells are those that produce antibodies (immunoglobulins). Memory cells are what their name implies—they act as a memory of previous antigen invasions and protect the body for many years from the antigen, e.g. tetanus or small pox (17,18,23).

T cells are also found in blood (80% to 85% of lymphocytes), lymph nodes, the thymus, and the spleen. They, too, produce subsets of cells. Generally, they assist B and other T cells by aligning antigens in proper order for destruction. There are memory cells in this group as well (18,19,23).

Antibodies

Numerous stimuli cause lymphocytes to produce antibodies. A number of antibodies, or immunoglobulins, circulate within the vascular systems and may deactivate antigens or tag them for later destruction. Immunoglobulin G (IgG) is the main immunoglobulin of the body; others include IgM, IgA, IgD, and IgE. All have rather specific duties within the immune system (17–19,23,29).

Summary

Anatomically, the lymphatic system consists of multiple channels that begin in the periphery of the body, run through a series of lymph nodes, and return lymph to the venous system. In the normal state, the lymphatic system equilibrates the flow of interstitial fluid and mediates the many immune elements for the protection of the internal systems.

References

1. Bartholinus, Th. De lacteis thoracis in homine brutisque nuperrime observatis. Copenhagen. Martzan M, 1652.
2. Hippocrates. *The Genuine Books of Hippocrates.* Adams F, trans. London: Sydenham Society; 1849.
3. *De Lactibus Siue lacteis venis Quarto Vasorum Mesaraicorum genere Nouo Inuento. Gasparis Aselli Cremon Is, Anatomici Ticinensis, Dissertatio.* Milan: Baptum Bidellium; 1627.
4. Foster M. *Lectures on the History of Physiology.* Cambridge: Cambridge University Press; 1901.
5. Choulant JL. *History and Bibliography of Anatomic Illustration.* Frank M, trans. and annot. New York: Hafner Publishing Company; 1934.
6. Rudbeck O. *Nova exercitation anatomica, exhibens ductus hepaticos aquosos et vasa glanularum serosa, nunc primum in venta, aeneisque figures delineate.* Vesteras: E Lauringer; 1653.
7. Fulton JF. The early history of the lymphatics with particular reference to Bartholin, Rudbeck, and Joliffe. *Bull Hennepin County Med Society.* 1938;9:5–10.
8. Harvey W. *Exercitatio anatomica de motu cordis et sanguini in animalibus.* Frankfurt: W Fitzer; 1628.
9. Wyall H. *William Harvey.* London: Parsons; 1924.
10. Hunter W. *Medical Commentaries.* No. 26. London: 1762.
11. Mascagni P. *Vasorum lymphaticorum corporis humani description et iconographi.* Siena: P Carli; 1787.
12. Picard J-D. *Lymphatic Circulation.* Lavaur, France: Editions Médicales Pierre Fabre; 1995.
13. Rouviere H. *Anatomy of the Human Lymphatic System.* trans. Tobias MJ, Ann Arbor, MI: MJ Edwards; 1938.
14. Sappey P. *Anatomie, physiologie, pathologie des vaisseaux lymphatiques consideres chez l'homme et les vertibres.* Paris: A Delahaye; 1874.

15. Kubik S. Zur Klinischen Anatomie des Lympsystesm, *Vehr Anat Ges*. 1975.

16. Bollinger A, Partsch H, Wolfe J, eds. *Initial Lymphatics, New Methods and Findings*. International Symposium; Zurich 1984. Stuttgart and New York: Georg Thieme Verlag; 1985.

17. Olszewski WL. *Peripheral Lymph: Formation and Immune Function*. Boca Raton, FL: CRC Press; 1985.

18. Weissleder H, Schuchhardt C, eds. *Lymphedema: Diagnosis and Therapy*. 3rd ed. Bonn: Kagerer Kommunikation; 2001.

19. Földi M, Kubik S, eds. *Lehrbuch der Lymphologie für Mediziner*. 5th ed Munich-Jena: Urban & Fisher; 2002.

20. Zhdanov DA. *General Anatomy and Physiology of the Lymphatic System*. Leningrad: Medgiz; 1952.

21. Kappert A, ed. *Lehrbuch und Atlas der Angiologie: Erkrankungen der Arterien, Venen, Kapillaren und Lymphgefässe*. 12th ed. Bern: Verlag Hans Huber; 1989.

22. Casley-Smith JR. Lymph and lymphatics. In: *Microcirculation*. New York: University Park Press; 1977; 1:421–430.

23. Kasseroller RG. *Compendium of Dr. Vodder's Manual Lymph Drainage*. Heidelberg, Germany: Haug; 1998.

24. Guyton AC, Granger HJ, Taylor AE. Interstitial fluid pressures. *Physiol Rev*. 1971.

25. Yoffey JM, Courtice FC. *Lymphatics, Lymph and Lymphoid Tissue*. London: Arnold; 1956.

26. Kubik S. *The Lymphatic System*. New York: Springer; 1985.

27. Olszewski WL, Engeset A. Immune proteins, enzymes, and electrolytes in human peripheral lymph. *Lymphology*. 1978;11:156–164.

28. Ryan TJ, Mallon EC. Lymphatics and the processing of antigen. *Clin Dermatol*. 1995;13(5):485–492.

29. Olszewski WL, Grzelak I, Ziolkowska A, Engeset A. Immune cell traffic from blood through the normal human skin to lymphatics. *Clin Dermatol*. 1995;13:473–483.

2
Differential Diagnosis of Lymphedema

Simon J. Simonian, Cheryl L. Morgan, Lawrence L. Tretbar, and Benoit Blondeau

Pathophysiology of Edema

As described in chapter 1, there is always fluid within the interstitial space, the space between tissue cells. The amount of fluid depends on 2 factors: the amount introduced into the interstitial space, and the amount removed from it. Fluid enters the space from arterioles and venules; some returns to the venules, and the remainder is taken up by the lymphatics. In the normal physiologic state, entrance and exit are approximately equal, so that tissues retain their usual morphologic appearance and function (1,2).

Edema (swelling) develops when the volume of interstitial fluid increases, either from increased inflow or decreased outflow, or both (3).

Lymphatic Causes of Edema

Primary Lymphedema

Primary lymphedema results when the lymphatics do not or cannot propel the lymph in adequate amounts, and the fluid sequesters within the interstitial or lymphatic spaces. It develops from an alteration or deficiency within the lymphatic collecting or transport systems. Primary lymphedema often occurs in the lower extremities, and affects women more than men (4–6). Many lymphatic malformations are described in chapter 4; a few are briefly reviewed below:

- Milroy disease (hereditary lymphedema type I) is a familial congenital disease and appears at or soon after birth (7,8) (Figure 2-1).

- Meige disease (hereditary lymphedema type II) develops later, e.g. at puberty, often after a minor injury, and causes foot and ankle swelling. Girls are affected more often than boys (9,10).
- Lymphedema praecox, another term for the 2 syndromes described above, has an early onset up to age 35 years (10,11).
- Lymphedema tardum is similar to praecox, but has an onset after age 35 years (10,11).
- Lymphangiomas are congenital, benign, often cystic malformations of the lymphatics and may be associated with other vascular malformations (4,12).

Secondary Lymphedema

Secondary lymphedema is swelling that follows some other incident or event, such as infection or injury (12,13).

Infection

- Filariasis, the most common cause of secondary lymphedema in the world, affects patients who have lived in or traveled in areas endemic with the disease; the worm's larvae migrate to the lymphatics, causing obstruction and damage (13,14) (Figure 2-2).
- Recurrent cellulitis, e.g. erysipelas, is acute and unilateral in the affected limb, often entering skin from a fungal skin infection (15,16).
- Lymphogranuloma venereum, a sexually transmitted disease, caused by chlamydia, often with enlarged inguinal lymph nodes.
- Scrofula, old term for tuberculous lymph nodes of the neck.

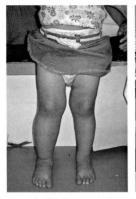
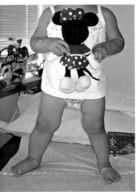

A

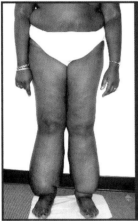
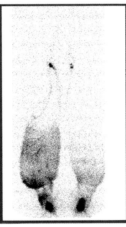

B

crystal absorption into the foot with lymphatic damage (Figure 2-3)

Cancer Treatment and Other Types of Trauma

- Any treatments, whether surgical or irradiation, can interrupt the normal flow of lymph, that results in the accumulation of lymph, i.e., lymphedema.
- Lymphadenectomy, or surgical excision of the inguinal, iliac, or auxiliary lymph nodes, the most common non-infectious cause worldwide, especially following breast cancer treatment, of chronic unilateral swelling (17).
- Nonsurgical trauma, e.g. radiation therapy to lymph node groups, may cause chronic unilateral swelling.
- Surgery of the prostate, uterus, or cervix may cause bilateral swelling.
- Recurrent and metastatic malignancy.
- Hodgkin and non-Hodgkin lymphoma.
- Reconstructive arterial surgery, e.g. saphenous vein harvest for coronary artery bypass

FIGURE 2-1. (A) An example of Milroy disease, the right leg of this 2-year-old baby has been swollen since birth. (B) This woman had mild swelling of the legs noted at age 10 years. The swelling was progressive until her lymphedema was finally diagnosed and treated at age 36. Dermal backflow is more prominent in the right leg, but is present in both (see Figure 2.8). The feet show the typical changes of lymphedema—swelling of the toes and feet, with deep flexion creases. (Photos courtesy Emily Iker.)

Inflammation

- Any of a group of non-infectious diseases causing edema, pain, or erythema.
- Systemic lupus erythematosus
- Rheumatoid arthritis, which may have combined muscle pump failure due to fixation and stiffening of the joints.
- Psoriatic arthritis
- Chronic dermatitis
- Retroperitoneal fibrosis
- Panniculitis
- Systemic diseases, e.g. Grave's disease, myxedema
- podoconiosis, elephantiasis caused by silica

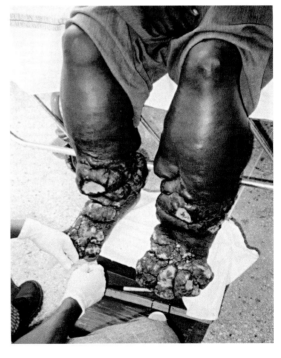

FIGURE 2-2. Filariasis, as seen in this man's legs, is endemic in Haiti and many other countries. (Photo courtesy CL Morgan.)

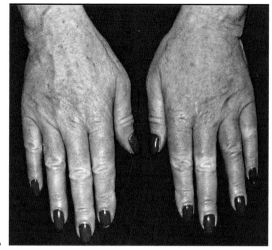

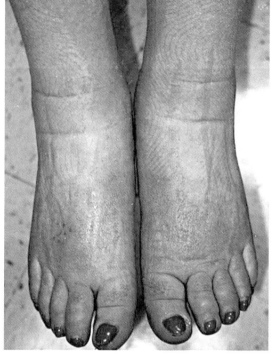

FIGURE 2-3. (A) Although the swelling in this patient's hands is mild, it nevertheless represents myxedema. (B) Her feet begin to show typical changes of lymphedema, with deepening of the flexion creases and swelling of the toes. (Photos courtesy CL Morgan.)

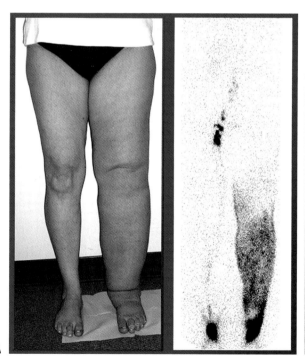

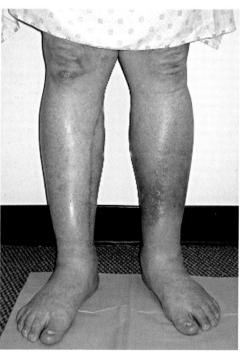

FIGURE 2-4. (A) This 46-year-old woman had surgery and radiation for uterine cancer. Lymphedema in her left leg is confirmed by the lymphoscintigram, which shows marked dermal backflow. (B) In another patient, the right greater saphenous vein was har-vested for a coronary artery bypass; lymphatic damage caused later lymphedema. Here the left leg shows the changes of chronic venous insufficiency with hyperpigmentation, slight edema, and hyperkeratosis. (Photos courtesy Emily Iker.)

- Factitious, self-inflicted trauma, e.g. constricting a limb with a rubber band to induce swelling (18).
- External injury to the body, e.g. an auto accident (Figure 2-4)

Other Causes of Edema

Chronic Venous Insufficiency

As explained in chapter 1, properly functioning venous and lymphatic systems help maintain a balance between interstitial and lymphatic fluid. A change in one system affects the other (12,19–22).

With venous disease in the legs, there is usually chronic damage to the veins and their valves. The result of valve failure is continuing reflux (backward flow of blood), increasing pressure on normal veins and damage to the surrounding tissues and lymphatic structures—chronic venous insufficiency (4,20,22). (See chapter 7 for more information.)

Hypoalbuminemia

Reduced blood concentration of proteins, especially albumin, reduces osmotic (oncotic) pressure and the reabsorption of interstitial fluid into the venous capillaries. Swelling is usually chronic, often bilateral (12,17).

- Excessive loss of albumin, glomerulonephritis, nephrotic syndrome, extensive burns.
- Malabsorption syndromes, inadequate absorption of protein, steatorrhea syndromes, protein calorie malnutrition, starvation, e.g. Kwashiorkor.
- Inadequate synthesis of albumin, cirrhosis, liver failure.

Drug-induced Edema

Several medications can cause or contribute to edema, complicating diagnosis (12,17,18). They include:

- hormones, estrogens, testosterone, corticosteroids, progesterone, and androgens
- antihypertensives, guanethidine, β-adrenergic blockers, calcium channel blockers, clonidine, hydralazine, methyldopa, minoxidil, reserpine, and labetalol

- nonsteroidal anti-inflammatory drugs, (NSAIDs)
- antidepressants, e.g. trazodone
- hypoglycemics, e.g. pioglitazone and rosiglitazone
- cytokines: GM-CSF, G-CSF, Il-4, Il-2, Interferon-a
- chemotherapeutics, e.g. cyclophosphamide, cyclosporine, mitramycin, and cytosine arabinoside
- antiviral, e.g. acyclovir

Differential Diagnosis of Edema

The differential diagnosis of edema requires a thorough historical review, physical examination, evaluation of treatment response, and occasionally special laboratory investigations. The examination report should include a diagram of the limb or affected area and standard measurements, e.g. limb circumference. Staging using these criteria is discussed in chapter 3.

Duration and Distribution

If the duration of the swelling is short, perhaps hours or days, and it is unilateral and painful, an acute process is suggested: deep vein thrombosis, cellulitis, abscess, ruptured Baker cyst, trauma, muscle compartment syndrome, ruptured gastrocnemius muscle, or reflex sympathetic dystrophy (12,18).

If the onset is gradual and progressive, over a period of weeks or months, and it is unilateral and painless, a chronic process is suggested: chronic venous insufficiency, post-thrombotic syndrome, lymphedema, (primary or secondary type), external venous compression, arteriovenous fistula, Klippel-Trenaunay syndrome, and soft-tissue or vascular tumors (12,17).

If the onset is gradual and progressive and swelling is bilateral, possible causes include: congestive heart failure, glomerulonephritis, the nephrotic syndrome, hypoproteinemia, drug reactions, cirrhosis of the liver, pretibial myxedema, constrictive pericarditis, lower limb dependency syndrome, lipedema, bilateral chronic venous insufficiency, bilateral lymphedema, or a malignancy in the pelvis, abdomen, or the retroperitoneal space. Advanced prostate carcinoma can cause lymphatic obstruction and bilateral leg edema, as can ovarian carcinoma or other pelvic tumors (12,17,18).

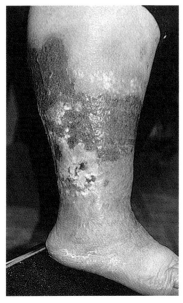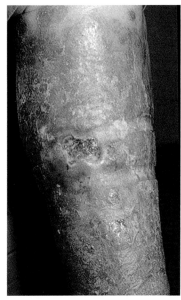

FIGURE 2-5. Superficial venous insufficiency caused these advanced cutaneous complications—edema, pigmentation, eczema, and ulceration. (Photos courtesy LL Tretbar.)

Dermatologic Changes

Skin changes are common with many types of swelling (22,23). They include:

- venous hypertensive pigmentation due to hemosiderin deposition, eczema, atrophie blanche (white atrophy), lipodermatosclerosis, or ulceration (Figure 2-5)
- taut skin, the inability to pinch a fold of skin at the base of the second toe (Kaposi-Stemmer sign), or prominent skin creases in the feet
- hyperkeratosis or papillomatosis (a warty skin texture)
- cellulitis, especially when recurrent (Figure 2-6)

Diagnostic Laboratory Tests for Systemic Disease

- The cardiopulmonary system is evaluated with chest x-rays, electrocardiograms, and echocardiograms.
- Kidney and liver functions are assessed with standard blood testing, which should include the blood albumin concentration.
- Thyroid function is also tested with standard blood tests, e.g. T3, T4.

Testing for Venous Disease

- different non-invasive and invasive tests are used to evaluate the veins for blood clots and function
- D-dimer, blood testing for deep vein thrombosis
- ultrasonographic imaging, to assess the deep, perforator, and superficial venous systems of the legs for evidence of old deep vein thrombosis and for the degree of valvular incompetence and reflux (Figure 2-7)
- contrast venography, to check for the presence of pelvic or abdominal thrombus
- computed tomography (CT) to check for pelvic pathology, especially malignancies and retroperitoneal fibrosis
- assessment of the ankle-brachial pressure index (ABPI), which is useful in determining arterial insufficiency in the legs of older patients and diabetics; compression therapy may worsen peripheral arterial disease.

Testing for Lymphedema

Lymphangioscintigraphy is the best laboratory test for lymphedema. A radioisotope-labeled colloid is injected into the web space between the

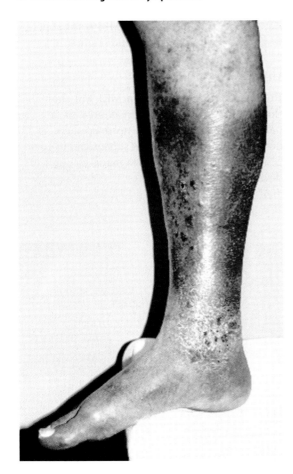

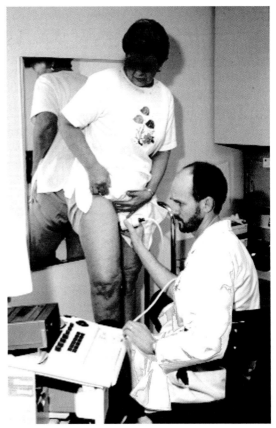

FIGURE 2-6. This man suffered a right deep vein thrombosis 12 years before this photograph was taken. There is marked hyperpigmentation, eczematoid changes in the calf with white atrophy, and small ulcerations on the ankle. Little edema had developed. (Photo courtesy LL Tretbar.)

FIGURE 2-7. Duplex ultrasonography is noninvasive, safe, and reproducible; it is relatively inexpensive and exhibits a high degree of accuracy. (Photo courtesy LL Tretbar.)

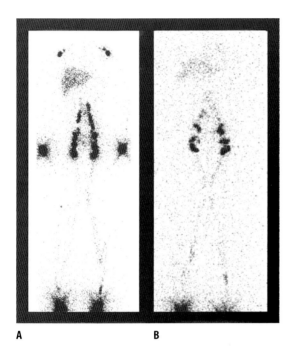

A   **B**

FIGURE 2-8. Lymphangioscintigraphy remains the basic test for assessing lymphatic function within the extremities. (A) This normal scan at 20 minutes demonstrates bilateral proximal flow of colloid that opacifies the inguinal, iliac, and axillary nodes and liver. (B) At 40 minutes, most of the tracer has dissipated. When the test is abnormal (see Figure 2-4), dermal backflow can be seen as the tracer leaks from the lymphatics. (Photos courtesy BB Lee.)

first and second toes. Using a gamma camera, the colloid movement is measured as it travels toward the proximal lymph nodes (24–26) (Figure 2-8). Slow progress of the radioisotope, compared with the normal lower limb, suggests hypoplasia of the peripheral lymphatics, as in primary lymphedema. If the radioisotope escapes from the main lymph channels, especially into the skin, it is called dermal backflow. This finding suggests lymph reflux, often seen in secondary lymphedema with proximal lymph obstruction.

Lymphangiography is another option that is rarely used today. This test uses radio-opaque lipiodol injected directly into a peripheral lymph vessel; x-rays monitor its proximal progress. This test is used for planning surgical lymphovenous anastomoses and for research purposes (27,28).

Both computed tomography (CT) and magnetic resonance imaging (MRI) show a typical subcutaneous honeycomb pattern in lymphedema, but not in other edemas. Of the 2, MRI is the superior test, as it also detects excess fluid (Figure 2-9).

Lipedema

In determining lipedema, an MRI will show that the soft-tissue swelling consists only of fat. The peripheral lymphatics are normal; there is no honeycomb appearance, and subcutaneous edema is absent. However, late lymphatic changes may develop (27) (Figure 2-10).

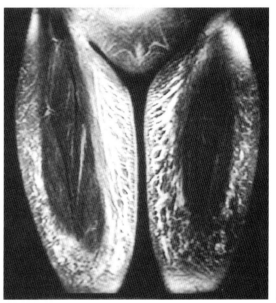

A

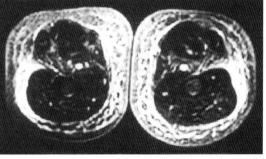

B

FIGURE 2-9. In the (A) sagittal view and (B) axial view of the lower extremities, an MRI shows an extensive honeycombed pattern in the soft tissue, a hallmark of chronic lymphedema not found in other edemas. Here the muscle compartment is unchanged, although it may be enlarged in the postthrombotic syndrome. MRIs can also provide quantitative assessment of lymphedema volume. (Photos courtesy BB Lee.)

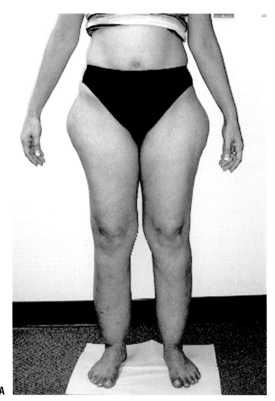

FIGURE 2-10. (A) Lipedema is characterized by a swelling of the hips and legs, but usually with none in the feet. In this case, a lymphoscintigram was normal. The fatty changes developed over a number of years; the feet are beginning to show lymphedematous changes, e.g. deep flexion creases and swelling of the dorsum and toes. (Photo courtesy Emily Iker.) (B) This woman's legs were normal until she had a car accident that traumatized them. The lipedema developed only in her legs; the torso and feet were spared. An ulcer that formed after a recent infection is seen on her left leg. (Photo courtesy CL Morgan.) (C) Diagnosis is difficult in this case: the feet are reasonably normal, but there are changes in the lower calves that suggest venous insufficiency. Extreme obesity is apparent as well, with a panniculus hanging below the patient's clothing. This patient deserves a complete evaluation that should include lymphangioscintigraphy. (Photo courtesy LL Tretbar.)

A

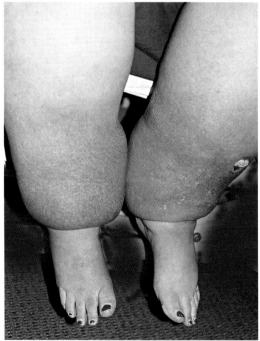

B

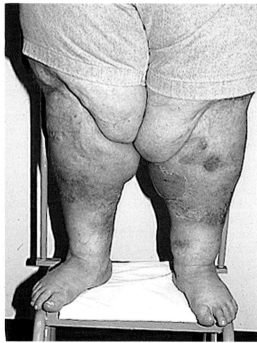

C

Summary

Information obtained from clinical and laboratory testing can help determine the probable cause of edema. Clinical evaluation with a thorough medical history is usually sufficient, as laboratory testing (e.g. lymphangioscintigraphy, MRI) is not always available. As accurate diagnosis is important, so that an appropriate treatment program can be planned and expectations of the treatment can be reviewed with the patient.

References

1. Drinker CK, Field E, Ward HK, Leigh OC. The composition of edema fluid and lymph in edema and elephantiasis resulting from lymphatic obstruction. *Am J Physiol.* 1934;109:572–586.
2. Ryan TJ, DeBerker D. The interstitium, the connective tissue environment of the lymphatic, and angiogenesis in human skin. *Clin Dermatol.* 1995;13(5):451–458.
3. Daroczy J. Pathology of chronic lymphedema. *Lymphology.* 1994;6:91–106.
4. Browse NL, Stewart G. Lymphoedema: pathophysiology and classification. *J Cardiovasc Surg.* 1985.
5. Olszewski WL. *Lymph Stasis: Pathophysiology, Diagnosis, and Treatment.* Boston: CRC Press; 1991.
6. Cluzan RV. Lymphatics and edema. In: Cluzan RV, Pecking AP, Lokiec FM, eds. *Progress in Lymphology XIII.* Amsterdam: Excerpta Medica, Elsevier Science; International Congress Series; 1992:716–717.
7. Nonne M. Vier Falle von Elephantiasis Congenita Hereditaria. *Virchow's Arch Pathol Anat.* 1891; 125(1):189–196.
8. Milroy WF. Chronic hereditary edema: Milroy's disease. *JAMA.* 1928;91:1172–1175.
9. Dale RF. The inheritance of primary lymphoedema. *J Med Genet.* 1985;22:274–278.
10. Kinmonth JB, Taylor GW, Tracy GD, Marsh JD. Primary lymphoedema. *Br J Surg.* 1957;45(189):1–9.
11. Wright NB. The swollen leg and primary lymphedema. *Arch Dis Child.* 1994;71:44–49.
12. Weissleder H, Schuchhardt C, eds. *Lymphedema: Diagnosis and Therapy.* 3rd ed. Bonn: Kagerer Kommunikation; 2001.
13. Dreyer G, Addiss D, Dreyer P, et al. *Basic Lymphoedema Management, Treatment and Prevention of Problems Associated with Lymphatic Filariasis.* Hollis, NH: Hollis Publishing; 2002.
14. Olszewski WL, Jamal S. Recurrent dermatolymphangioadenitis (DLA) is responsible for progression of lymphedema. Progress in Lymphology XV. *Lymphology.* 1996;(Suppl.)29:331–334.
15. Herpertz U. Lymphödem und Erysipel. *Lymph-Forsch.* 1998.
16. Blumberg H, Janig W. Clinical manifestation of reflex sympathetic dystrophy and sympathetically maintained pain. In: Wall P, Melzack R, eds. *Textbook of Pain.* Edinburgh: Churchill Livingstone; 1993.
17. Földi M, Kubik S, eds. *Lehrbuch der Lymphologie für Mediziner.* 5th ed. Munich-Jena: Urban & Fisher; 2002.
18. Browse N, Burnand K, Mortimer P, eds. *Diseases of the Lymphatics.* London: Arnold; 2003.
19. Blondeau B, Helling TS, Morgan, CL. Insuffisance veineuse et obesité. *Phlebologie.* 2003;56.
20. Klippel M, Trenaunay P. Du naevus variqueux osteohypertrophique. *Arch Gen Med.* 1900;185:641–672.
21. Tretbar LL. *Venous Disorders of the Legs.* London: Springer-Verlag; 1999.
22. Partsch H, Urbanek B, Wenzel-Hora B. Dermal Lymphangiopathie ei chronisch venoser Insuffizienz. In: Bollinger A, Partsch H, eds. *Initiale Lymphstrombahn-Internationales Symposium.* Zurich: Thieme; 1984:205–209.
23. Ramelet AA, Monti M. *Phlebologie.* 2nd ed. Bonn: Kagerer Kommunikation; 1993;22:238–239.
24. Stemmer R. Ein klinisches Zeichen zur Früh-und Differentialdiagnose des Lymphodems. *Vasa.* 1976; 5(3):261–262.
25. Pecking A, Cluzan R, Desprez-Cureley A. *Indirect lymphangioscintigraphy in patient with limb edema.* In: Heim L, ed. Immunology and Hematology Research Foundation; 1984;3(4):327–328.
26. Weissleder H, Weissleder R. Lymphedema: evaluation of qualitative and quantitative lymphangioscintigraphy in 238 patients. *Radiol.* 1988;167(3):729–735.
27. Hummel E, Weissleder H. Lymphgefasse bie Lipodem. In: Clodius L, Baumeister RGH, Foldi E, eds. *Lymphologica.* Munich: Medikon; 1989;16: 89–98.
28. Picard J-D. *Lymphatic Circulation.* Lavaur, France: Editions Médicales Pierre Fabre; 1995.

3
Classification and Staging of Lymphedema

Cheryl L. Morgan and B.B. Lee

Introduction

Although there have been numerous international attempts to classify and stage lymphedema, there is no single method that provides a comprehensive view of the disease that defines its etiopathophysiology or describes the significant overlap between the recorded stages. Not only is the process of classification and staging deficient, it is confusing to many physicians because the definitions and terminology differ widely.

Therefore, the authors propose a method of staging that includes the spectrum of identifiable disease processes, defined not only by physical changes but also by their etiopathophysiology. Further, an improved method of staging should coalesce research, and help advance educational programs for the health professionals.

This chapter presents some of the controversial aspects of current staging methods and a new proposed staging system for lymphedema. However, until a consensus is reached for the adoption of a more standardized approach, the current staging systems may be used.

Condition

When evaluating a swollen limb or tissue, first its condition, the general type of change in the tissue, is described. This may be a cursory look at the swelling, or a more specific and thorough description of the overall changes that cause it to differ from the normal limb or tissue. One traditional idea is that lymphedema is a simple accumulation of fluid or lymph in the tissues; we now know, however, that the development of lymphedema represents a dynamic, actively changing process. Chronic lymphedema can no longer be considered a benign, static condition, but is a progressive and degenerative disease (1,2). This demands that all changes in the tissues be acknowledged, not just the swelling.

The importance of accurate staging is obvious—without proper intervention at the appropriate time, the condition is destined to develop serious complications (3). Improved classification and staging standards can better identify these complications and determine the most useful interventions, all of which depend on the general health, age, and medical history of the patient.

Classification

Currently, the classification of lymphedema is defined by the origin of the condition, i.e. primary or secondary (4). It must be remembered that classification of lymphedema is not a staging technique. This system (of classification) is used internationally and meets the authors' present expectations.

Primary Lymphedema

Simply defined primary lymphedema results from any deficiency of proper lymphatic development that cannot be attributed to injury, trauma, illness, treatment, or disease, e.g. medication, radiation, or phlebolymphedema (4–6).

Depending on the patient's age when clinical symptoms manifest, primary lymphedema has traditionally been classified into 2 groups: lymphedema praecox becomes evident early, and up until age 35 years; lymphedema tardum develops at or after age 35. There is some suspicion that lymphedema tardum may be a secondary lymphedema; often there is little evidence of congenital defects to ascertain its etiology (4,6) (see chapter 4).

Primary lymphedema can also be categorized as congenital or hereditary forms. Hereditary forms are familial and may be traced. The congenital form represents a birth defect in the lymphatic system caused by a genetic abnormality during embryogenesis. Using this classification, the true congenital type is limited to only a fraction of primary lymphedemas that are apparent at birth. Not all lymphedemas presenting at birth are a consequence of a genetic abnormality (7); lymphedematous defects can be secondary to traumatic events during pregnancy.

To further confound the issue, not all congenital lymphedemas are clinically detectable at birth but may manifest later. These variations in presentation make it difficult, if not sometimes impossible, to classify the involvement of the affected body part (6,8,9).

Secondary Lymphedema

Secondary (acquired) lymphedema can result from many external factors that alter, both anatomically and functionally, an otherwise normal lymph-conducting system (6,10). Identifying the exact cause of the swelling is the most important part of the diagnostic investigation. Eight causative factors are usually considered (11–15): trauma, malignancy, venous disease, infection, inflammation, immobility, parasites, and factitious conditions.

Because several causes of secondary lymphedema can be treated, with a reasonable chance of recovery, no effort should be spared in this critically important part of chronic lymphedema management. Proper etiologic identification and treatment may also halt the progression of the

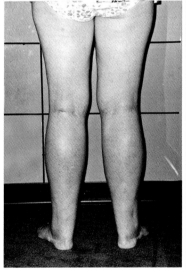 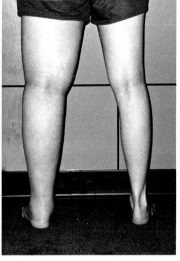

A   B

FIGURE 3-1. (A) This represents a secondary stage I lymphedema. The edema recedes with elevation and there are no other physical problems. Bilateral stripping of the saphenous veins for varicosities in this 36-year-old woman caused enough lymphatic damage to the stripping sites that lymphedema developed. Note the loss of the Achilles space and the hyperemia of the legs. Four weeks of complete decongestive therapy reduced the distal symptoms, and the patient continued home self-care. (B) A case of primary lymphedema, stage 1. [Both images (A and B), are photographs taken at initial evaluation.] Primary lymphedema is present in the right leg of this 15-year-old girl, whose symptoms appeared at age 12 with the onset of menses. (Photographs courtesy of CL Morgan.)

disease; there is no cure for an already damaged lymphatic system. All lymphedemas should be considered secondary until proven otherwise (13,14).

Obviously, significant ambiguities exist in the diagnosis of primary and secondary lymphedemas. Unfortunately, the present classification and staging systems fail to clarify them. Therefore, an advanced staging system can assist in proper diagnosis.

Staging

Once an etiologic diagnosis of lymphedema is established, staging based on clinical manifestations is mandated. Staging provides a reasonably objective system recording abnormalities and plays an essential role in the planning of appropriate medical intervention and in determining the effectiveness of the intervention. New staging strategies should provide more definitive categorization of the disease, based on the degree and severity of anatomic and physiologic changes (Figures 3-1 to 3-3) (15,16).

Staging of any disease process should accomplish at least 5 primary goals:

1. Evaluate and identify the distinctive characteristics of the condition, e.g. possible etiology and symptoms.
2. Determine the duration, extent, and severity of the disease.
3. Outline appropriate medical intervention and expected outcomes.
4. Help patients understand their disease, possible management options, and anticipated results, and promote adherence to recommended treatment.
5. Help insurance companies ascertain the possible expenses necessary to obtain the anticipated outcome.

Current Staging Methods

The *Consensus Document on the Diagnosis and Treatment of Peripheral Lymphedema* was first published in 1995 by the International Society of Lymphology (ISL) and updated in 1998 following the ISL Congress held in Madrid the prior year (17). However, neither document mentioned staging. The first description of staging was in the revised ISL Consensus Document of 2001, published in *Lymphology* that same year (17). The staging was enumerated as follows:

Stage I represents an early accumulation of fluid relatively high in protein content (when compared with venous edema), and which subsides with limb elevation.

Stage II occurs when limb elevation rarely reduces tissue swelling and pitting is manifest. As tissue fibrosis supervenes late in stage II, the limb may or may not pit.

Stage III encompasses lymphostatic elephantiasis, in which the skin does not pit, and trophic skin changes such as acanthosis, fat deposits, and warty overgrowths develop.

The severity of each stage is based on volume differences: minimal, <20% increase in limb volume; moderate, 20% to 40% increase in limb volume; severe, >40% increase in limb volume.

The most recent revision of the ISL Consensus Document (2003) describes 4 stages of lymphedema, based on risk, local skin changes, and the severity and degree of edema (17). This revision includes stage 0, described as a latent or subclinical condition where swelling is not evident despite impaired lymph transport. It may exist months or years before overt edema occurs. Many lymphologists contend that stage 0 represents only the risk of developing lymphedema and may create difficulty with insurance coverage and inappropriate expectations for future treatment planning (18).

The 2003 Consensus Document is the document most referred to in publications. It is incorrect to identify it as the staging system endorsed by the ISL; the document itself states, ". . . a more detailed and inclusive classification needs to be formulated in accordance with understanding of the pathogenic mechanism of lymphedema" (17).

A few examples of staging systems used across the globe are presented here to illustrate the complexities involved and the need for standardization to adequately address various issues, from diagnosis to intervention.

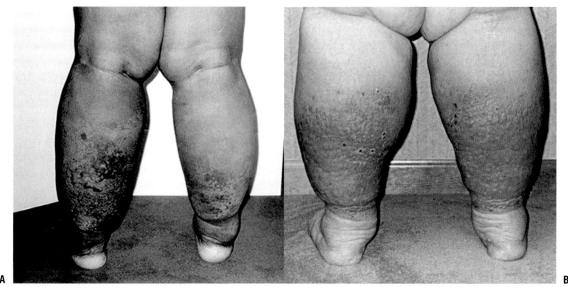

A   B

FIGURE 3-2. (A) This 52-year-old woman presented with a history of swelling of approximately 7 years, 9 pregnancies, and diabetes. Venous studies reveal moderate reflux in both saphenous veins. Edema is not reduced with elevation, significant fibrosis is evident, and 3 to 4 episodes of cellulitis per year have been reported for the past 3 years. This lymphedema is considered stage II and secondary to venous insufficiency under the current ISL system. (B) Complica-tions of diabetes and obesity experienced by this 61-year-old woman have led to 8 hospitalizations for cellulitis in the past 22 months. She has reported symptoms since she was 9 years old that suggest primary lymphedema, and that her mother and sister have "heavy legs." Extensive fibrosclerosis is present, and distally the skin will no longer pit with pressure. (Photographs courtesy of CL Morgan.)

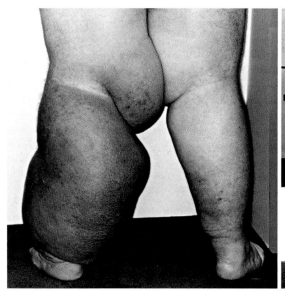

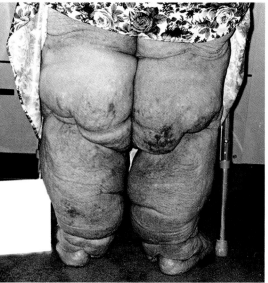

A   B

FIGURE 3-3. (A) This is an example of stage III lymphedema sec-ondary to surgery and radiation for melanoma. This 38-year-old male presents with significant volume increase of the left leg, mul-tiple hospitalizations for cellulitis, and recent disability from the size and weight of the limb. Symptoms presented immediately after groin dissection. Postradiation, the swelling involved the genitalia, and 6 months later the right leg began to swell. (B) This 67-year-old woman presented with massive lymphedema of both lower extremities, which she reports she has had since childhood. Unable to ambulate, dress, bathe, or transfer without assistance, she has recently experienced 3 episodes of cellulitis and recurrent skin breakdown. Distally, the edematous tissues are nonpitting, with significant trophic changes, including acanthosis and multiple skin folds. (Photos courtesy of CL Morgan.)

Földi Method of Staging

For years the Földi staging system has been the predominant method of classification among European and American clinicians. In recent publications, it too has included a stage 0 (14). The stages are detailed as follows:

Stage 0, latency: asymptomatic, focal fibrosclerotic tissue changes, diagnosis by lymphangioscintigraphy.

Stage I, spontaneously reversible: high-protein edema; focal fibrosclerotic tissue alterations; pitting edema reduced by elevation; possible "pain of congestion"; diagnosis by basic procedures.

Stage II, spontaneously irreversible: extensive fibrosclerosis; proliferation of adipose tissue; brawny hard swelling not reduced with elevation; diagnosis by basic procedures.

Stage III, elephantiasis: extensive fibrosclerosis (as with stage II); proliferation of adipose tissue, invalidism; diagnosis by basic procedures.

Pitting Edema Scale

Pitting edema refers to an indentation of the skin that occurs when simple finger pressure is applied. If the skin can pit, the inference is that the onset of swelling is recent and therefore less serious. Edema is not detectable clinically until the interstitial fluid volume reaches 30% above normal (19). The pitting edema scale is detailed as follows:

1+ edema is barely detectable
2+ a slight indentation occurs with pressure and remains momentarily
3+ a deeper impression occurs, but skin returns to normal within 5 to 30 seconds
4+ the impression remains more than 30 seconds

Nonpitting edema is present when pressure is applied but no indentation occurs. This suggests that more advanced subcutaneous tissue changes have developed and fluid cannot be displaced with mere pressure. Although this manual measuring technique has been replaced by more objective and reliable measuring devices, like the tonometer, it is still widely used by physicians and health care professionals.

Staging by Limb Size

As simple as it is to measure the diameter of the limbs, there is significant concern by health professionals that this system does not adequately represent the patient's true condition. It does not, for example, provide for the evaluation of lymphedema of the trunk or other parts of the body, nor does it indicate the duration of the disease process, the development of skin changes, or other important considerations required for planning management and determining outcome results (20). Staging by limb size is determined as follows:

Mild: less than 3 cm differential between affected and unaffected limbs
Moderate: 3 to 5 cm differential between affected and unaffected limbs
Severe: more than 5 cm differential between limbs

All of these examples of staging are internationally adapted, as indicated in the chapter's introduction. These attempts by health care professionals to modify the current methods described above are indicative of a need for change. This further complicates communications with patients or insurance companies in describing the severity, treatment options, outcomes, and length of treatment usually required to achieve the goals.

In many of the staging models, the values assigned to each stage primarily describe complications of changes in tissues of affected limbs (20,21). These changes range from lymphoceles, fistulas, vesicles, chylous reflux, skin folds, and eczemas, to sepsis, infections, and chronic wounds. Described as knobs, bumps, protuberances, blisters, sclerosing panniculitis, lipodermatosclerosis, or mossy foot, all are manifestations of impaired lymphatics that present differently but are not well described in literature or medical reference materials (21).

Staging by Clinical Symptoms

Clinical evaluation is the most common method used to diagnose and stage lymphedema, since laboratory tests are too expensive or simply not available. This particular staging system addresses specific changes in the lower extremities of patients with lymphedema secondary to parasitic infections. It was developed by physicians and the research team for the Lymphatic Filariasis Prevention and Treatment Program in Recife, Brazil (12). (Another, completely different scale identifying only 4 stages was devised by the Brazilian Society of Lymphology [22]).

Staging by clinical symptoms is detailed as follows:

Stage I: swelling increases during the day, and disappears overnight

Stage II: swelling does not go away overnight; occasional infections; may have entry lesions

Stage III: persistent edema; beginning of shallow skin folds; occasional infections

Stage IV: persistent edema; presence of skin knobs, protrusions, and bumps; occasional infections

Stage V: persistent edema; the presence of 1 or more deep skin folds; occasional infections

Stage VI: mossy lesions develop on the skin surface; numerous deep skin folds; frequent infections

Stage VII: unable to perform daily activities; numerous deep skin folds and skin lesions present; frequent infections

The method developed by the Italian Society of Lymphangiology (Campisi-Michelini) provides further example of the diverse clinical symptom staging systems (22). The stages are detailed as follows:

Stage I: no edema in an at-risk patient (preclinical)

Stage II: edema that reduces spontaneously with elevation and during the night

Stage III: edema that does not reduce spontaneously and only partially with treatment; recurrent episodes of lymphangitis

Stage IV: fibrotic edema; disappearance of tendon and bone shapes

Stage V: elephantiasis complicated with relapsing skin infections, with involvement of deep layers (muscles, joints)

Location, Volume, Fibrosis Scale

To clarify the degree to which lymphedema is manifested beyond standard volumetric measurements, Austrian physicians Kasseroller and Brenner developed the location, volume, fibrosis (LVF) scale (23). This approach can help to identify and collect data that can be numerically represented and allows progress to be tracked more effectively. This tool is not a method of staging lymphedema, but is one that quantifies 3 elements of the condition most often focused on in treatment plans. This scale could be used in conjunction with staging lymphedema to provide clear data that can be followed to measure improvement (Table 3-1).

Similar to the Clinical Etiologic Anatomic Pathologic (CEAP) classification for the symptomology of chronic venous disease, it is not as complex to employ, and its objectives are clear (24). The objectives are to more easily identify the method of treatment most effective, present patients with expected outcomes, and provide insurance carriers with measurable data and criteria to determine reasonable reimbursements for each case.

Proposed Staging of Lymphedema

To compensate for deficits of the numerous staging methods, the authors propose modifying the ISL stages into a more specific 4-stage system. Acknowledging that lymphangioscintigraphy is not consistently available or used for diagnosis, the 4-stage system would permit both clinical assessment and laboratory data to define the stage (2). However, establishing a fourth stage with quantification of symptoms and correlated treatment options necessitates an aggressive educational program for physicians, to help them prescribe and monitor the patients' treatments and outcomes. This expanded staging method can be helpful in selecting treatment options, determining clinical results, evaluating the progress of the disease for the patient and health professional, and predicting risk, especially as insurance companies determine policy coverage. The proposed stages are defined as stages I to IV.

Clinical Staging

Clinical factors are based primarily on the condition of the skin and subcutaneous soft tissues found with subjective and objective evaluation;

TABLE 3-1. Location, volume, fibrosis scale (LVF).

Location: Axilla			Inguinal		Volumetric Increase		Fibrosis	
S	Left	S	Left	V0	1.00–1.05	F0	<1.25	
D	Right	D	Right	V1	1.05–1.10	F1	1.25–2.00	
L1	Trunk	L1	Trunk	V2	1.10–1.25	F2	2.00–3.50	
L2	Lower arm	L2	Calf	V3	1.25–1.50	F3	>3.50	
L3	Lower arm & hand	L3	Calf & foot	V4	>1.50	F4	+ color changes	
L4	Upper & Lower arm	L4	Calf & thigh	—	—	F5	+ secondary complications	
L5	Entire arm	L5	Entire leg	—	—	—	—	
L6	Hand	L6	Foot	VX	Not defined more precisely			
		LX	+ Genitals					

From Kasseroller RG, reference 23.

the severity of skin changes and the degree of dermatofibrosclerosis are especially important (14,16).

Other conditions are scored independently: local, and/or systemic infection, limitation of daily activities (ADL) by subjective symptoms that include pain, sensory complaints (heaviness, tightness, numbness), and difficulties in sleeping, performance of work, domestic duties, or recreational activities (Table 3-2).

Functional limitations comprising measurable physical factors such as the strength of an affected limb, the volume of edema, limitation of range of motion (e.g. brachioplexus), and restricted mobility (e.g. wheelchair bound) are objective reports considered in this method (14,21).

A separate laboratory staging, based on lymphangioscintigraphy findings, complements the clinical findings. The lymphoscintigraphic findings are also divided into 4 stages, I to IV.

Laboratory Staging: Lymphangioscintigraphy

Laboratory staging is based on the lymphangioscintigraphy findings observed initially and throughout the course of treatment. These repeatable tests help determine the effectiveness of treatment or possible progression of the disease (25) (Table 3-2).

Combining careful clinical staging with laboratory evaluation has greatly improved the diagnostic capabilities, especially in difficult situations. These 2 systems appear to provide better predictability of treatment outcomes and support more

rational decision making for potential surgical intervention (2,5,11).

When lymphangioscintigraphy is not available, values can be established for other available tests, such as magnetic resonance imaging (MRI) or computed tomography (CT) scanning (26–28). The results do not necessarily alter the treatment approach. The 4 stages are based on the number of findings in each of the clinical and laboratory factors. This system can meet many requirements of health professionals and significantly aid in the amalgamation of research.

A fourth stage helps identify cases that may prove unresponsive to therapies, e.g. patients with multiple comorbidities, limited functional capacity, frequent infections, and could indicate when surgical intervention might provide better results for the patient's quality of life (14,22).

Quality of Life

Quality of life measurements are a vital inclusion in the diagnosis and treatment of lymphedema (29). They are equally useful during the course of treatment, but because they are too subjective to standardize, a simplified scale can be used. An example is provided below (see Table 3-3). As an adjunct measurement, it helps determine the impact of the disease on the patient, family members, work or social settings, and ultimately the patient's ability to cope with the condition (29,30). A quality of life assessment can also help determine the effectiveness of contemporary management methods (31). It is the authors' experience that utilizing a quality of life tool assists in

TABLE 3-2. Clinical staging and laboratory staging (lymphoscintigraphic staging).

Clinical	Laboratory
Stage I Edema (swelling): mild and/or easily reversible (+) Skin changes: none without dermatofibrosclerosis (DFS) (−) Sepsis (systemic and/or local): none (−) Function limitations (FL): none (−) Daily activity limitation (ADL): no limitation (−)	**Stage I** Lymph node uptake (LN): decreased (±) Dermal backflow (DBF): none (−) Collateral lymphatics (CL): good visualization (+) Main lymphatics (ML): decreased visualization (±) Clearance of radioisotope from injection site (CR): decreased lymphatic transport (±)
Stage II Edema: moderate and/or reversible with effort (+) Skin changes: none to minimal without DFS (±) Sepsis: none to occasional (±) Function limitations (FL): mild to moderate (+) ADL: occasional and/or moderate limitations (±)	**Stage II** Lymph node uptake (LN): decreased to none (−) Dermal backflow (DBF): visualization (+) IIA: extent of DBF does not exceed 1/2 of each limb IIB: exceeds 1/2 of each limb CL: decreased visualization (±) ML: poor to no visualization (±) CR: greater decrease (±)
Stage III Edema: moderate to severe and/or minimally reversible to irreversible (±) to (−) Skin changes: moderate with significant DFS (+) Sepsis: common (+) less than 4 times a year Function limitations (FL): moderate to significant (+) ADL: frequent and significant limitations (+)	**Stage III** Lymph node uptake (LN): decreased to none (−) Dermal backflow (DBF): visualization (+) CL: poor visualization (−) ML: no visualization (−) CR: no clearance (−)
Stage IV Edema: severe and/or irreversible (−) Skin changes: severe with advanced DFS (+) Sepsis: very frequent (+) more than 4 times a year Function limitations (FL): moderate to severe (+) ADL: constant and severe limitations (+)	**Stage IV** Lymph node uptake (LN): none (−) Dermal backflow (DBF): poor to no visualization (−) CL: no visualization (−) ML: no visualization (−) CR: no clearance (−)
Clinical stage is established with a composite of 3 or more findings.	*Laboratory stage is established with a minimum of 2 or more lymphoscintigraphic findings.*

BB Lee, CL Morgan, J Bergan. Findings: (+) present, (−) Absent, (±) Either : both

TABLE 3-3. Quality of life scale.

Excellent 5 points	No limitation of daily activity or difficulty on extra activity (e.g. hobbies) physically, psychologically, and/or socioeconomically
Good 3 points	Some limitation on extra activity occasionally physically, psychologically, and/or socioeconomically, but with no limitation to daily activity
Fair 1 point	Significant limitation on extra activity but no limitation on daily activity physically, psychologically, and/or socioeconomically, or occasionally some limitation on both daily and extra activity.
Poor −1 point	Significant limitation on both daily activity and extra activity, frequently physically, psychologically, and/or socioeconomically
Bad −3 points	Profound limitation on daily activity as well as extra activity or no feasible daily activity without assistance physically, psychologically, and/or socioeconomically

BB Lee, J Bergan. Lymphology 2005:38(2).

promoting adherence with the treatment plan, thus improving the outcome of treatment.

Outcome Measurements

The patient's response to treatment must be monitored both during and after the treatment program. Outcome measurements are based on the improvement of clinical and laboratory evaluation (31–33).

Assessment of the clinical response to treatment relies on subjective improvement of symptoms, e.g. pain, discomfort, and fatigue, and on evidence of objective improvement, e.g. reduction of swelling, improved range of motion of joints, and elimination of sepsis. These combined findings are used to assign the appropriate stage and thereby determine the effectiveness of treatment

(32). Improvement of the quality of life can be added separately to the final evaluation.

When progression of the disease is arrested by the treatment program, as determined by the new clinical and laboratory staging, the result is categorized as "excellent." If there is no progression of the disease, but moderate clinical improvement, a "good" result is recorded. When there is minimal progression of the disease, with or without clinical improvement and an unchanged clinical staging, the result is "fair." If there is steady progression of the disease and simultaneous clinical deterioration, the response is "poor."

When more conservative methods fail to provide desired results, the new staging criteria should identify this situation and provide the opportunity to evaluate the possible use of surgical therapies. This new clinical staging, based on new clinical criteria, appears to be more precise than the current ISL staging or its modifications. It can be used by physicians for laboratory diagnosis, or by therapists who can use clinical findings to establish a tentative diagnosis (33). Either assessment can determine the proper stage for documentation and insurance purposes.

Summary

Although fully functional, the proposed staging system can be improved. As it attempts to include the entire spectrum of related medical and non-medical factors in the staging process, it itself requires continuous evaluation. For example, establishing other criteria for testing methods, e.g. MRI, CT, or bioimpedence, would make it more universal and more compatible with other staging methods. A prospective and periodic review of the testing techniques and the information obtained by them is essential for long-term improvement (34).

The goal is to improve patient care by improving the evaluation of the patient and his or her disease. These collective data can help establish more accurate staging that in turn will allow more accurate intervention at the appropriate time.

This is only possible when the medical community is willing to form a consensus on:

- defining a common diagnostic and treatment language

- creating a more universal vocabulary of terms
- improving the investigation, collection, and reporting of patient information
- maintaining consistency in research, documentation, and publication
- developing new educational opportunities for the health professional

With all concerned health providers working together to achieve these, this goal is not only possible, but also obtainable.

References

1. Nieto S. Stages of lymphedema according to correlation among pathophysiology, clinical features, imaging, and morphology of the affected limbs. *Lymphology.*

2. Lee BB, Bergan JJ. New clinical and laboratory staging systems to improve management of chronic lymphedema. *Lymphology.* 2005;38:122–129.

3. Olszewski WL. *Lymph Stasis: Pathophysiology, Diagnosis and Treatment.* Boston: CRC Press; 1991.

4. Kinmonth JB. *The Lymphatics: Diseases, Lymphography and Surgery.* London: Arnold; 1972.

5. Bruna J, Miller AJ, Beninson J. The clinical grading and simple classification of lymphedema. *Lymphology.* 2002;35.

6. Weissleder H, Schuchhardt C. *Lymphedema: Diagnosis and Therapy*, 2nd ed. Bonn: Kagerer Kommunikation, 1997.

7. Kinmonth JB, Taylor GW, Tracy GD, Marsh JD. Primary lymphoedema. *Br J Surg.* 1957;45(189): 1–10.

8. Casley-Smith JR. The pathophysiology of lymphoedema. In: Heim LR, ed. IXth International Society of Lymphology. Tel Aviv, Israel Immunology Research Foundation, Newburgh, USA, 125–130.

9. Browse NL, Stewart G. Lymphoedema: pathophysiology and classification. *J Cardiovasc Surg.* 1985;26:91–106.

10. Daroczy J. Pathology of chronic lymphoedema. *Lymphology.* 1995;28(3):151–158.

11. Weissleder H, Schuchhardt C, eds. *Lymphedema: Diagnosis and Therapy.* 3rd ed. Bonn: Kagerer Kommunikation; 2001.

12. Dreyer G, Addiss D, Dreyer P, et al. *Basic Lymphoedema Management, Treatment and Prevention of Problems Associated with Lymphatic Filariasis.* Hollis, NH: Hollis Publishing; 2002.

13. Olszewski WL, Jamal S. Recurrent dermatolymphangioadenitis (DLA) is responsible for progression of lymphedema. Progress in Lymphology XV. *Lymphology.* 1996;(Suppl.)29:331–334.

14. Földi M, Kubik S, eds. *Lehrbuch der Lymphologie für Mediziner*. 5th ed. Munich-Jena: Urban & Fisher; 2002.

15. Browse N, Burnand K, Mortimer P, eds. *Diseases of the Lymphatics*. London: Arnold; 2003.

16. Stemmer R. Ein klinisches Zeichen zur Früh-und Differentialdiagnose des Lymphodems. *Vasa*. 1976;5(3):261–262.

17. International Society of Lymphology. The diagnosis and treatment of peripheral lymphedema. Consensus Document of the International Society of Lymphology. *Lymphology*. 2003;36:84–91.

18. International Congress of Lymphology. Consensus Meeting on Staging Lymphedema, Salvador, Brazil, 2005.

19. Mortimer PS. Managing lymphedema. *Clin Exp Dermatol*. 1995;13(5):499–505.

20. Földi E, Földi M, Weissleder H. Conservative treatment of lymphedema of the limbs. *Angiology*. 1985;36(3): 171–180.

21. Lee BB, Kim DI, Hwang JH, et al. Contemporary management of lymphedema—personal experiences. *Lymphology*. 2002;38(1):28–31.

22. International Congress of Lymphology. Salvador, Brazil, 2005.

23. Kasseroller RG. LVF—Lymphödemklassifikation des inguinal und axillären Tributargebeites. *Journal für Lymphologie* 2. Jhg. 2/2002:2–7.

24. Labropoulus N. CEAP in clinical practice. *Vasc Surg*. 1997;31.

25. Pecking A, Cluzan R, Desprez-Cureley A. Indirect lymphangioscintigraphy in patient with limb edema. Progress in lymphology. Proceedings of 9th internation congress; Tel Ariv. 1985;201–206.

26. Weissleder H, Weissleder R. Lymphedema: evaluation of qualitative and quantitative lymphangioscintigraphy in 238 patients. *Radiol*. 1988;167(3): 729–735.

27. Yeo YC, Lee ES, Lee BB. Ultrasonographic evaluation of lymphedema. *Ann Dermatol*. 1997(9):126.

28. Picard J-D. *Lymphatic Circulation*. Lavaur, France: Editions Médicales Pierre Fabre; 1995.

29. Azevedo WF, Boccardo F, Zilli A, et al. A reliable and valid quality of life in patients with lymphedema—version of the SF-36. *Lymphology*. 2002; 35(1):177–180.

30. McWayne J, Heiney SP. Psychologic and social sequelae of secondary lymphedema: a review. *Cancer*. 2005;104:457–466.

32. De Godoy JMP, Braile DM, et al. Quality of life and peripheral lymphedema. *Lymphology*. 2002;35(2): 44–45.

33. Choi JY, Lee KH, Kim SE. Quantitative lymphoscintigraphy in post-mastectomy lymphedema: correlation with circumferential measurements (abstract). *Korean J Nucl Med*. 1997;31.

34. Hwang JH, Kwon JY, Lee BB, et al. Changes in lymphatic function after complex physical therapy for lymphedema. *Lymphology*. 1999;32(1):15–21.

4
Lymphatic Malformation

B.B. Lee

Lymphatic malformation is the most common form of congenital vascular malformation and may exist alone or with other vascular malformations, e.g. lymphovenous malformations (1–4).

To clarify these differences, at the Hamburg consensus meeting of 1988 the International Society for the Study of Vascular Anomaly divided lymphatic malformations into 2 groups: the truncular form, and the extratruncular form (5,6).

Although both forms are the consequence of genetic arrest, the arrest occurs at different stages of lymphangiogenesis. This difference is important when planning appropriate interventions.

When developmental arrest occurs at an early stage of embryogenesis, it remains in the extratruncular form; when arrest occurs at a later stage of angiogenesis, it becomes the truncular form (7,8).

Because the lymphatic arrest of the extratruncular form occurs at an earlier stage of embryogenesis than the truncular form, it retains many unique characteristics of its evolutionary potential. Accordingly, given the appropriate stimuli, e.g. trauma, surgery, hormones, or pregnancy, its lesions can continue to grow (9).

The primitive evolutionary potential of the extratruncular form may cause difficulty in management—for example, an ill-planned treatment strategy for lesions like cystic or cavernous lymphangioma may provoke recurrences (2).

Truncular Forms

Primary Lymphedema

Primary lymphedema represents the truncular form of lymphatic malformation and is frequently considered a separate disease, although its close relationship with the extratruncular form is not always appreciated. Nor is its close tie to other forms of congenital vascular malformations fully recognized. Because of its clinical presentation, it is often grouped with secondary lymphedema as chronic lymphedema (10,11).

In contrast, the truncular form does not possess an evolutionary potential, because its defect occurs at a later, more mature stage of development. Other alterations in structure and function develop: ectasia, aplasia, hypoplasia, and hyperplasia of lymph nodes and the lymph-collecting system. Depending on their severity, the defects create lymphodynamic changes that are manifested clinically as chronic lymphedema, (2,12–14) (Figure 4-1).

Diagnosis

Diagnostic investigation of the swollen limb is initiated with a carefully taken history and complete physical examination. These clinical examinations may be adequate to make an appropriate diagnosis. If not, they should be followed by noninvasive diagnostic tests designed specifically to assess the truncular form, from a simple tape measurement of the limb to infrared optometric determination of limb volume.

When available, lymphoscintigraphy (see chapter 2) should be used to assess lymphatic function within the extremities (15–17). It also evaluates the degree and extent of anatomic truncular form involvement throughout the collecting and conducting systems and the lymph nodes (18).

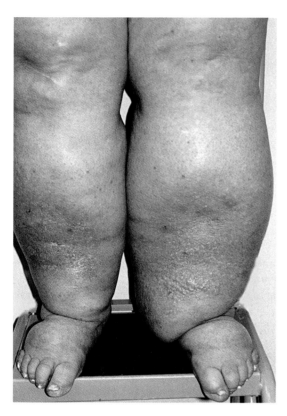

FIGURE 4-1. This image coveys the essence of advanced primary lymphedema. The swelling developed during this woman's adolescent years and continued until it was treated in her early 20s. The calves are enormous and show cutaneous changes of hyperpigmentation and hyperkeratosis. The feet show the typical signs of lymphedema, with swollen toes with deepening flexion creases. CDT-based treatment was successful, and the patient was able to live a relatively normal life. (Photo courtesy LL Tretbar.)

Magnetic resonance imaging (MRI) and computed tomography (CT) scanning are occasionally added, e.g. for quantitative assessment of lymphedema volume. Newly developed ultrasonographic and MR lymphangiography may be considered before treatment plans are fully developed (1,2).

An investigation of the extratruncular form may be warranted during clinical evaluation of the truncular form, to rule out simultaneous involvement. The remainder of the differential diagnosis is outlined in chapter 2. In addition to evaluation of the lymphatic system, the superficial and deep venous systems must be assessed for patency and function with duplex ultrasonography.

Management

When developing management strategies, a multidisciplinary team is essential; this can minimize morbidity and prevent an improper approach to this lifelong medical challenge (19).

A program of complete decongestive therapy (CDT) that includes manual lymphatic drainage, wrapping, exercise, and skin care should initiate the clinical management of truncular-form lymphatic malformations (20,21). Sequential, intermittent, pneumatic compression may be added in selected cases.

Surgical intervention should be considered only if medical treatments have failed during the earliest possible stages of lymphedema (4). Fortunately, a number of reconstructive surgical procedures are available (4,10,22–25). Multiple lymphovenous microsurgical anastomoses (24,25) can be performed if the primary lymphedema is caused by lymph node dysplasia alone. Free lymph node transplant (4,26) can also be performed for lymph node dysplasia, especially when dysplasia is combined with inadequate lymph-collector development.

The free-graft technic transplants the harvested lymph node groups to the recipient site; it requires an end-to-end anastomosis of donor artery and vein to recipient vessel. It is therefore unavailable to those patients receiving lympho-venous anastomotic reconstruction.

Outcome Assessment

Follow-up assessment by the multidisciplinary management team is recommended on an average of every 6 months (4,10). This includes a clinical and basic laboratory evaluation that looks for subjective improvement of symptoms, as well as objective evidence of physical improvement (see chapter 5). Where available, lymphoscintigraphic evaluation should be included on an annual basis for patients with truncular forms of lymphatic malformations, regardless of treatment type (18).

The author included MR and/or ultrasonographic lymphangiography in the postoperative evaluation. Both tests are still in the investigative stage for assessing the clinical results of reconstructive, venolymphatic anastomotic, or free lymph node transplantation.

Candidates for ablative (excisional) surgery are those who, in the later stages of lymphedema, develop grossly disfigured limbs that cannot be effectively treated by conventional conservative methods (27–29) (see chapter 6). The addition of surgical therapy might improve the response of conservative management for the truncular form; however, experience thus far has been too limited to draw any reliable conclusions for long-term synergistic effects.

Extratruncular Forms

Depending on the severity of the clinical presentation, the extratruncular forms of lymphatic malformations are grouped as lymphangioma, and lymphangiomatosis. They are different from lymphangiosarcoma (30–33).

Lymphangiomas (34–36) are hamartomatous and neoplastic tumors of different sizes. They are embryonic tissue remnants that usually behave independently from other malformations. They may occasionally communicate with a normally developed lymph-conducting system but seldom interfere with normal functions.

Depending upon the size and the ability of the embryonic tissue remnant to hold lymph fluid, lymphangiomas are further divided into 3 groups: lymphangioma simplex, lymphangioma cavernosa, and cystic lymphangioma (hygroma). Here the term "hygroma" is identified more specifically as cystic hygroma, which has become synonymous with lymphangioma (37).

These forms are entirely different from lymphangiectasia of the lymph-conducting system, which is a simple ectatic change within the lymph-collecting vessels; it usually belongs to the truncular form, which includes aplasia, hypoplasia, and hyperplasia.

Diagnosis

The diagnosis of this extratruncular form of lymphatic malformations is made with noninvasive and invasive tests (1,2). The diagnostic testing is used to differentiate it from other extratruncular forms, especially from combined vascular defects and hemolymphatic malformations.

Usually the diagnosis can be made without invasive tests. Ultrasonography (38), lymphoscin-tigraphy, MRI, and CT are the basics for the initial diagnostic workup (39). More esoteric tests—such as Tc-99m RBC whole-body blood pool scintigraphy (WBBPS) (40) and transarterial lung perfusion scintigraphy (TLPS), using Tc-99m macro aggregated albumin (41)—are occasionally indicated.

If the relationship of the lymphangioma with the lymph-conducting system is unclear, ascending or percutaneous direct puncture lymphography or bipedal lymphography, using lipiodol-based contrast material, should be considered.

Management

In general, cavernous lesions are more likely to develop postoperative lymph fistulae. An attempt to control the skin vesicles with superficial therapies, e.g. laser, electrocautery, or diathermy, is destined to fail. It provides only temporary relief, because the vesicular lesion maintains an elevated contractile pressure and can rupture.

Once the extent and degree of tissue involvement is established, the multidisciplinary team should select the lesions that require therapy first. Treatment priority should be given to lesions located near vital organs or structures that might threaten critical functions, including respiration, vision, hearing, or eating. Early treatment should also be considered for lesions with accompanying complications, lymph leakage, hemorrhage, or recurrent infections. Other candidates for early treatment include those with symptomatic lesions, with or without cosmetically severe deformities or functional disability, e.g. hand, foot, wrist, and ankle (1,2,34–37) (Figure 4-2).

Fortunately, the extratruncular form of lymphatic malformation generally is less serious than other forms of congenital vascular malformation, e.g. venous or arteriovenous malformations. They rarely become a life- or limb-threatening condition. In contrast to limbs with arteriovenous malformations, a conservative approach has been accepted for managing the extratruncular form of lymphatic malformation (1,2).

Definitive treatment of children's problems should be deferred until the child attains a level of development that diminishes the risk of therapy. Should complications develop, such as acute respiratory or alimentary embarrassment,

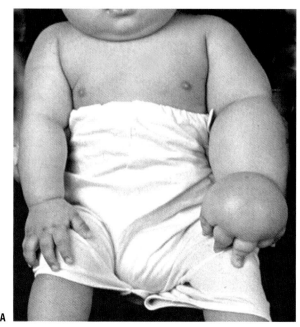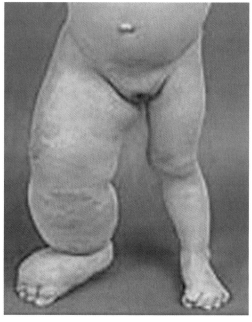

A   B

FIGURE 4-2. (A) Like this child, candidates for early treatment are those with severe functional disability. (B) Early aggressive management is warranted when normal function is seriously compromised. Here skin lesions are already apparent on this child's right leg.

emergency life-saving measures may be required, especially in neonatal and young pediatric patients.

Sclerotherapy

Sclerotherapy is usually preferred as the initial treatment and entails the injection of a solution that irritates the tissues and causes them to sclerose (collapse). It is often adequate treatment, but should it fail, excision of deep-seated subcutaneous or submucous extratruncular lesions may be indicated (1,2).

As recurrence following sclerotherapy is common, we recommend a less vigorous agent, OK-432, as the first choice for sclerotherapy (42,43). OK-432 is a lyophilized exotoxin of the low-virulence Su strain of type III group A Streptococcus pyogenes. It may be less effective than more powerful agents, like ethanol, but diminishes the risk of complications.

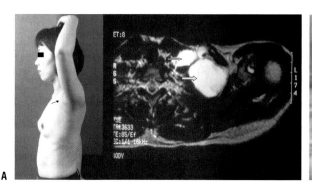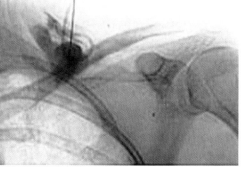

A   B

FIGURE 4-3. (A) From the surface, a mild swelling appears along the left upper anterior chest wall and subclavicular region. It represents the extratruncular form of lymphatic malformation.

(B) Deeper macrocystic lesions, often known as cystic lymphangiomas, were treated successfully with direct percutaneous-puncture OK-432 sclerotherapy.

Even if sclerotherapy fails, it does more good than harm if subsequent excision is necessary; it thickens the wall of a single-layer endothelial lesion and permits an easier dissection than with a primary thin-walled lesion.

Multicystic, lobulated lesions are ideal candidates for sclerotherapy alone, but require multiple injection sessions. Unfortunately, it is virtually impossible to inject the sclerosant into microsize cavernous lesions. In addition, these honeycombed lesions are more likely to communicate with the normal lymphatic system, thereby risking injury from sclerosant leakage to perilymphatic tissues, such as nerves and blood vessels. Published research has shown that OK-432 is safer than other sclerosant, even when leakage occurs. Multisession OK-432 sclerotherapy can be performed as an independent therapy, mainly to cystic lesions, with remarkable results (Figure 4-3).

Sclerotherapy with absolute alcohol (ethanol) should be reserved for select cases, e.g. recurrent or failed OK-432 sclerotherapy cases (1,2).

Another common sclerosant, sodium tetradecyl sulfate, has also been used for closure of congenital cystic lesions, but its long-term efficacy has yet to be determined.

In our published clinical trials, ethanol, when used as a sole treatment modality to recurrent or deeply seated lesions—preferably the cystic types—gave excellent results. Superficial lesions treated independently with OK-432 also responded well in most cases. Cavernous lesions, when treated independently, generally do not respond well. When possible, cavernous extratruncular lesions were treated with pre- and perioperative sclerotherapy combined with surgical excision; however, the results of this approach were mixed and of limited success.

Excision

Certain lesions, e.g. neck lesions that extend into the deep mediastinal structures, require surgical excision because of their massive size and extensive involvement. Even so, the risk of injury to adjacent vessels and nerves is great during dissection; injury may result in potentially life-threatening conditions, especially in a young age group (34–37).

Although there is no optimal time for surgical excision, it is safer to defer an extensive dissection or excision as long as possible. Partial excision of an easily accessible lesion is acceptable as the first part of a multistage approach; it allows a better chance for a later excision of the residual lesion. Emergency operations should be limited to decompressive surgery designed to relieve acute symptoms until a later, more elective opportunity is available (34–37).

This extratruncular lesion of lymphatic malformation is rarely life threatening, in contrast to other vascular malformations, such as arteriovenous malformations. When one encounters a lymphatic malformation lesion adherent to a vital structure, it is better to accept incomplete excision rather than to risk possible damage to the vital structure—a crucial difference from the management of venous or arteriovenous malformations.

Complete excision provides the only possible cure for the extratruncular form of lymphatic malformations. Nevertheless, incomplete excision and recurrence are present in more than 50% of cases because of anatomical or technical difficulty, especially in the neonatal and pediatric group. Complications, such as skin flap necrosis and post-excisional cosmetic disfigurement, disillusion many surgeons.

Recurrence is a critical issue, as the extratruncular form of lymphatic malformation retains the original characteristic of the mesenchymal cell, i.e. the pluripotential to regrow its original tissue (1,2) (Figure 4-4).

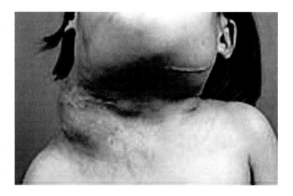

FIGURE 4-4. Following ill-planned surgery, recurrent massive swelling is pervasive along the right incisional scar. The soft tissue lesions of this child's neck extended into the retropharyngeal and left submandibular region, and necessitated further excisional surgery to relieve vital functions for breathing and swallowing.

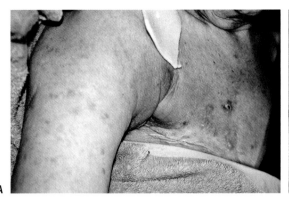
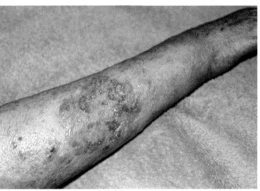

A   B

FIGURE 4-5. (A) Although infrequent, patients with lymphangio-sarcoma may present themselves to treatment centers. This person was treated with chemotherapy and radiation that improved the condition of her arm and chest. (B) Local swelling in the arm was treated with manual lymph drainage and compression. (Photo courtesy CL Morgan.)

Outcome Assessment

Treatment results are based on findings of subjec-tive and objective clinical improvement: pain, fluid leakage, infection, and reduction of lesion size or swelling. Both clinical and laboratory assessment may be necessary. The results are graded as "excellent" when the treated lesion has disappeared completely, "good" when there is sub-stantial reduction or nearly complete disappear-ance of the lesion, and "fair" for moderate improvement.

Evaluation of the extratruncular form should be made every 6 months by the team; in addition to clinical assessment, duplex ultrasonography and MRI may be needed as well.

Lymphangiosarcoma

Primary lymphedema has an inherent risk, however slight, of developing a malignancy—lym-phangiosarcoma derived from the chronically inflamed lymphedematous tissue (30,31). It is the only malignant disease that develops in the lymphatic system and is often known as Stewart-Treves sarcoma. Although lymphangiosarcoma is an extremely rare complication of primary lymphedema, the possibility of its development cannot be ignored.

It starts as painless, reddish-purple skin nodules that steadily increase in size and number. Because of its rarity, it is invariably neglected or misdiag-nosed as a common skin disorder. Ulceration, bleeding, and infection complicate the process that eventually spreads throughout the body; at that time, it is usually too late for a cure.

When discovered early, however, a combination of radiation therapy, intravenous, and intra-arterial chemotherapies can effect temporary relief or remission—a better alternative than palliative amputation (32,33). Once the diagnosis is confirmed, an extensive investigation should be performed to determine the extent of metastasis, and whether an aggressive treatment program is justified (Figure 4-5).

Lymphangioma Circumscriptum

Lymphangioma circumscriptum is a rare extra-truncular lesion that requires special attention to determine the extent of connective tissue involvement with deeper tissues. Masquerading as benign lesions in different sizes and colors, mul-tiple vesicular lesions develop on the skin and mucous membranes. Their appearance may be misleading, because the process involves transder-mal penetration of the cavernous extratruncular lesions into subdermal, submucosal, or subcuta-neous tissues. High contractile pressure vesicula-tion of the surface tissues may cause rupture (Figure 4-6).

Transdermal or transmucosal communications, causing visible skin or mucosal lesions, must be eradicated before other treatment is begun.

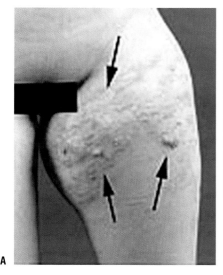

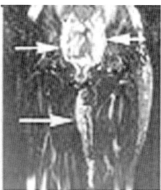

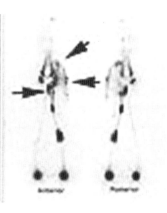

B

A

FIGURE 4-6. (A) Here lymphangioma circumscriptum is visible with its seemingly benign lesions appearing in different sizes and colors on the skin and mucous membranes. (B) Penetration into pelvic structures was confirmed by MRI; lymphoscintigraphy showed extensive dermal backflow.

It must be shown that a communication does not exist between the lesion and adjacent lymph-conducting systems. The lesions should be assessed by appropriate methods, such as ultrasonography or MRI.

Lymphangiomatosis

Diagnosis

Lymphangiomatosis is defined as a "diffuse, infiltrating type of extratruncular form of lymphatic malformation" by the Hamburg classification system. Subcutaneous and skeletal lesions dominate this vascular malformation. Although lymphangiomatosis is rare, it presents a challenge to the clinician who has managed the simpler lesions of cystic or cavernous lymphangiomas and now must manage these extensive subcutaneous and skeletal lesions.

Part or the entire limb may be involved; the subcutaneous lesions present as a diffuse swelling, exhibit an extensive involvement throughout the limb, and create a striking physical appearance.

Spongiform lymphangiomatosis shows fluid movement that shifts according to elevation or position of the limb, a phenomenon found in other vascular malformations of the lower extremity.

Skeletal lymphangiomatosis, an extratruncular lesion involving the bone, may manifest itself as an independent disease without evidence of concomitant soft tissue involvement. It too deserves a full investigation. X-ray findings of demineralized bone may mimic other demineralizing diseases: distant malignant metastatic lesions, multiple myeloma, hyperparathyroidism, polyostotic fibrous dysplasia, or metabolic lipid disease.

Lymphangiomatosis deserves a complete investigation to determine the possibility of other organ involvement. An evaluation should include the visceral and skeletal systems using CT/MRI of the abdomen and mediastinum, whole-body lymphoscintigraphy with delayed and interval evaluation, and percutaneous direct-puncture lymphangiography.

Management

The management of lymphangiomatosis, depending on the extent of involvement, is relatively straightforward and similar to that of other extratruncular lesions—sclerotherapy and surgical excision. Unfortunately, pathological long bone fractures are frequent during the growing age and

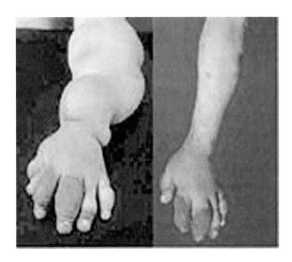

FIGURE 4-7. Lymphangiomatosis extends the length of this child's forearm and fingers and showed both macro- and microcystic lesions (left). Complete resection of the microcystic lesions followed preoperative OK-432 and ethanol sclerotherapy to the macrocystic lesions (right).

may cause devastating outcomes with severe disability. New multidisciplinary approaches must be found to improve the treatment results of these complex lesions (Figure 4-7).

Hemangioma

Congenital vascular malformations are frequently called capillary or cavernous hemangiomas by clinicians and histopathologists, even though a congenital vascular malformation is entirely different from a genuine infantile-neonatal hemangioma (44,45).

Originating from proliferative endothelium, hemangiomas are the most common vascular tumor to arise during infancy. They appear during fetal or early neonatal life and are characterized by rapid initial growth followed by spontaneous regression during later childhood (46).

A true peripheral congenital vascular malformation, however, comprises a group of birth defects that develop in various peripheral vascular systems, following developmental arrest in various stages of embryonic life. In contrast to hemangiomas, in which increased mitotic activity is often observed, a congenital vascular malformation is not hypercellular but is composed of normal mature endothelium.

The congenital vascular malformation is usually recognizable at birth, grows commensurate with the child, has a tendency to expand through puberty, and unlike a hemangioma does not regress.

Proper differentiation between the 2 vascular problems is mandatory. Each requires a different treatment strategy, even though they belong to the same category of vascular anomalies (47).

Lymphovenous Malformation

Klippel-Trenaunay Syndrome

Klippel-Trenaunay syndrome is the most common combined form of congenital vascular malformations—lymphovenous malformations embodied within a larger group of hemolymphatic malformations (2,48–51). Klippel-Trenaunay syndrome is not an inherited disorder, although it is congenital. Earlier reports, including the original paper by Klippel and Trenaunay, failed to recognize the lymphatic component, which produces many of the edema symptoms.

In contrast to the older eponym-based terminology, the Hamburg method classifies Klippel-Trenaunay syndrome as a venolymphatic malformation. This terminology provides a clue to its etiology, anatomy, and pathophysiology. The new classifications are based on the "predominant component" of the chronic vascular malformations and refer to the specific vascular system affected by the developmental arrest (5,6).

A triad of symptoms characterizes Klippel-Trenaunay syndrome (50,51): cavernous hemangioma (port-wine stain); bone and limb hypertrophy (52,53), which develop in most cases; and varicose veins that appear in about three-quarters of the patients. Approximately 65% of patients have the 3 tissue changes. It is sometimes called the angio-osteohypertrophy syndrome, and females are affected approximately twice as often as males (52,53).

Port-wine stains, often appearing on the lateral leg, are caused by dysplastic vasculature. Varicose veins are common and extensive. Although the greater saphenous vein is usually spared congeni-

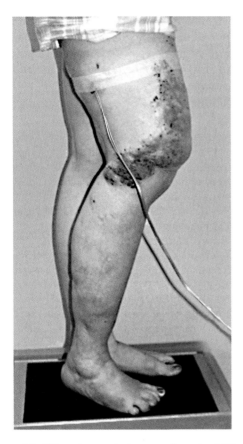

FIGURE 4-8. This patient made her own diagnosis of Klippel-Trenaunay syndrome, having reviewed her symptoms on the Internet. During this examination, a flat Doppler probe determines the direction and velocity of blood flow in the lateral thigh vein. Duplex ultrasonography was also performed to further delineate the status of the venous system. The discrepancy in her leg length suggests vascular bone involvement. A port-wine nevus completes the triad of symptoms. (Photo courtesy LL Tretbar.)

involvement, e.g. liver, lungs, kidneys, or large intestine, may produce complications, such as spontaneous rupture of hemangiomas and internal bleeding. Other complications of Klippel-Trenaunay syndrome include skin ulceration, cellulitis, deep vein thrombosis, and pulmonary embolism.

Parkes Weber Syndrome

Diagnosis

Arteriovenous fistulae are rarely found in the extremities of Klippel-Trenaunay syndrome patients. They are, however, the primary feature distinguishing Klippel-Trenaunay syndrome from the Parkes Weber syndrome (54). The absence of fistulae and the presence of low-velocity venous malformations suggest a diagnosis of Klippel-Trenaunay syndrome, rather than Parkes Weber syndrome.

With an improved understanding of theses syndromes, we must recognize the different truncular and extratruncular forms and consider their contributions to the pathophysiologic process. For example, the extratruncular forms present in venolymphatic malformations will exert their pluripotential characteristics originating from the embryologic mesenchymal cells. The truncular forms, however, will only exert hemodynamic changes on the venous and lymphatic vascular systems and on the bony and soft tissues as well.

Treatment

Treatment should be directed at specific physiological problems. In the truncular form—for example Klippel-Trenaunay syndrome—the embryonic lateral marginal vein is frequently excised or sclerosed to arrest severe reflux and progressive venous insufficiency.

In contrast, lymphangioma, an extratruncular form of lymphatic malformation, is seldom sited for treatment except to control complications, lymph leakage, intralesional bleeding, or sepsis. As with other primary lymphedemas, the truncular form of lymphatic malformations—such as aplasia, hypoplasia, hyperplasia of lymph

tal alteration, the deep veins may be valveless, aneurysmal, or absent. A large lateral marginal thigh vein often serves the limb as its major venous outflow conduit. Lymphedema develops from these vascular changes, notably in the legs, and is treated in a fashion similar to that for other primary lymphedemas (Figure 4-8).

Osteoarticular changes may present in only 1 leg and evolve during the first 5 years of life. They include soft tissue and bony hypertrophy, which may cause postural deformities and spinal scoliosis (53).

Lymphangiomas are less common, but they may accentuate other lymphatic changes. Visceral

collecting vessels and lymph nodes—is treated with CDT-based conservative treatment.

The interrelationships among the multiple vascular malformations are complex. Their interactions often create unpredictable, adverse responses to each other, either by their natural presence or in the treatment.

Genetic Prospects

Although presently handled as separate entities, the truncular and extratruncular forms of lymphatic malformations may need to be combined especially for the future treatment strategy; they are the result of the same developmental genetic deficit, although occurring at different stages of differentiation.

Recently, new genetic research has suggested that gene therapy holds promise for the treatment of lymphatic malformations within the fields of angiogenesis and vasculogenesis (55). Although the feasibility for therapeutic implementation of gene therapy to lymphatic malformation is far from reality, there is vigorous pursuit of the genetic possibilities.

The correction of defective lymphangiogenesis would be beneficial for contemporary management of lymphangioma, as well as for primary lymphedema.

Exogenous growth factor administration would open a new chapter for effective gene and gene-product therapy. Recently, it was confirmed that "Anti-VEGFR-3 neutralizing antibody" seems to completely halt lymphatic vascular regeneration. Therefore, a "molecular antidote" to the pathological overgrowth of lymphangiomatosis could become a major force that creates a chance for a cure in the near future (56).

Recognition of this enormous potential for contemporary management has caused some lymphologists to alter their approach to the treatment of lymphatic malformations.

Summary

During a period when lymphologists are increasingly aware of the complexity of vascular malformations, they are using newer methods of classification and improved testing technology to plan treatments more specific to the lesions' pathophysiology. Many treatment modalities are under re-evaluation for inclusion in the therapist's armamentarium; they can provide an increasingly individualized and effective approach to these difficult problems.

References

1. Lee BB. Lymphedema-angiodysplasia syndrome: a prodigal form of lymphatic malformation (LM). *Phlebolymphology*. 2005;47:324–332.
2. Lee BB, Seo JM, Hwang JH, et al. Current concepts in lymphatic malformation (LM). *Vasc Endovascular Surg*. 2005;39:67–81.
3. Jacob AG, Driscoll DJ, Shaughnessy WJ, et al. Klippel-Trenaunay syndrome: spectrum and management. *Mayo Clin Proc*. 1998.
4. Lee BB. Current issue in management of chronic lymphedema: personal reflection on an experience with 1065 patients. (Commentary). *Lymphology*. 2005;38.
5. Belov ST. Anatomopathological classification of congenital vascular defects. *Semin Vasc Surg*. 1993.
6. Belov S. Classification, terminology, and nosology of congenital vascular defects. In: Belov ST, Loose DA, Weber J, eds. *Vascular Malformations*. Reinbek, Germany: Einhorn-Presse; 1989.
7. Bastide G, Lefebvre D. Anatomy and organogenesis and vascular malformations. In: Belov ST, Loose DA, Weber J, eds. *Vascular Malformations*. Reinbek, Germany: Einhorn-Presse; 1989.
8. Woolard HH. The development of the principal arterial stems in the forelimb of the pig. *Contrib Embryol*. 1922.
9. Lee BB. Critical issues on the management of congenital vascular malformation. *Ann Vasc Surg*. 2004;18:380–392.
10. Lee BB, Kim DI, Hwang JH, et al. Contemporary management of chronic lymphedema—personal experiences. *Lymphology*. 2002;35.
11. Lee BB. Chronic lymphedema, no more stepchild to modern medicine. *Eur J Lymphology*. 2004;14:6–12.
12. Mortimer PS. The pathophysiology of lymphedema. *Cancer*. 1998.
13. Papendieck CM. Lymphangiomatosis and dermo-epidermal disturbances of lymphangioadenodysplasias. *Lymphology*. 2002;35.
14. Wolfe JH, Kinmonth JB. The prognosis of primary lymphedema of the lower limbs. *Arch Surg*. 1981.
15. Williams WH, McNeill GC, Witte MH, et al. Evaluation of peripheral lymphedema by longitudinal lymphangioscintigraphy. *Lymphology*. 2002;35.

16. Olszewski WL. Lymphoscintigraphy helps to differentiate edema of various etiologies (inflammatory, obstructive, posttraumatic, venous). *Lymphology*. 2002;35.

17. Bernas MJ, Witte CL, Witte MH. The diagnosis and treatment of peripheral lymphedema. *Lymphology*. 2001.

18. Lee BB, Bergan JJ. New clinical and laboratory staging systems to improve management of chronic lymphedema. *Lymphology*. 2005;38:122–129.

19. Lee BB, Bergan JJ. Advanced management of congenital vascular malformations: a multidisciplinary approach. *Cardiovasc Surg*. 2002;10:523–533.

20. Casley-Smith JR, Mason MR, Morgan RG. Complex physical therapy for the lymphedematous leg. *Int J Angiol*. 1995;4:134–142.

21. Hwang JH, Kwon JY, Lee BB, et al. Changes in lymphatic function after complex physical therapy for lymphedema. *Lymphology*. 1999;32.

22. Baumeister RGH, Siuda S. Treatment of lymphedemas by microsurgical lymphatic grafting: what is proved? *Plas Reconstr Surg*. 1990.

23. Campisi C, Boccardo F, Zilli A, et al. Long-term results after lymphatic-venous anastomoses for the treatment of obstructive lymphedema. *Microsurgery*. 2001.

24. Krylov V, Milanov N, Abalmasov K. Microlymphatic surgery of secondary lymphoedema of the upper limb. *Ann Chir Gynaecol*. 1982.

25. Olszewski WL. The treatment of lymphedema of the extremities with microsurgical lympho-venous anastomoses. *Int Angiol*. 1988.

26. Becker C, Hidden G, Godart S, et al. Free lymphatic transplant. *Eur J Lymphol*. 1991;6:75–80.

27. Homans J. The treatment of elephantiasis of the legs. *N Engl J Med*. 1936.

28. Kim DI, Huh S, Lee BB, et al. Excision of subcutaneous tissue and deep muscle fascia for advanced lymphedema. *Lymphology*. 1998;31.

29. Auchincloss H. New operation for elephantiasis. *P R J Public Health Trop Med*. 1930.

30. Wysocki WM, Komorowski A. Stewart-Treves syndrome. *J Am Coll Surg*. 2007;205(1):194–195.

31. Laguerre B, Lefeuvre C, Kerbat P, et al. Stewart-Treves syndrome arising in post-traumatic lymphedema. *Bull Cancer*. 1999.

32. Goetze S, Schmook T, Audring H, et al. Successful treatment of Stewart-Treves syndrome with liposomal doxorubicin. *J Dtsch Dermatol Ges*. 2004.

33. Lans TE, de Wilt JH, van Geel AN, et al. Isolated limb perfusion with tumor necrosis factor and melphalan for nonresectable Stewart-Treves lymphangiosarcoma. *Ann Surg Oncol*. 2002.

34. Alqahtani A, Nguyen LT, Flageole H, et al. Twenty-five years' experience with lymphangiomas in children. *J Pediatr Surg*. 1999.

35. Al-Salem AH. Lymphangiomas in infancy and childhood. *Saudi Med J*. 2004.

36. Orvidas LJ, Kasperbauer JL. Pediatric lymphangiomas of the head and neck. *Ann Otol Rhinol Laryngol*. 2000.

37. Stromberg BV, Weeks PM, Wray RC Jr. Treatment of cystic hygroma. *South Med J*. 1976.

38. Lee BB, Mattassi R, Choe YH, et al. Critical role of duplex ultrasonography for the advanced management of a venous malformation (VM). *Phlebology*. 2005.

39. Lee BB, Choe YH, Ahn JM, et al. The new role of MRI (magnetic resonance imaging) in the contemporary diagnosis of venous malformation: can it replace angiography? *J Am Coll Surg*. 1984.

40. Lee BB, Mattassi R, Kim BT, et al. Contemporary diagnosis and management of venous and AV shunting malformation by whole body blood pool scintigraphy (WBBPS). *Int Angiol*. 2004.

41. Lee BB, Mattassi R, Kim BT, et al. Advanced management of arteriovenous shunting malformation with transarterial lung perfusion scintigraphy (TLPS) for follow-up assessment. *Int Angiol*. 2005;24: 173–184.

42. Ogita S, Tsuto T, Deguchi E, et al. OK-432 therapy for unresectable lymphangiomas in children. *J Ped Surg*. 1991;26.

43. Kim KH, Kim HH, Lee BB, et al. OK-432 intralesional injection therapy for lymphangioma in children. *J Korea Asso Ped Surg*. 2001.

44. Mulliken JB. Cutaneous vascular anomalies. *Semin Vasc Surg*. 1993.

45. Mulliken JB, Glowiczki J. Hemangiomas and vascular malformations in infants and children: a classification based on endothelial characteristics. *Plast Reconstr Surg*. 1982.

46. Mulliken JB, Zetter BR, Folkman J. In vivo characteristics of endothelium from hemangiomas and vascular malformations. *Surg*. 1982.

47. Lee BB. Statutes of new approaches to the treatment of congenital vascular malformations (CVMs)—single center experiences [editorial review]. *Eur J Vasc Endovasc Surg*. 2005;30:184–197.

48. Klippel M, Trenaunay J. Du noevus variqueux et osteohypertrophique. *Arch Gén Méd*. 1900.

49. Servelle M. Klippel and Trenaunay's syndrome. *Ann Surg*. 1985.

50. Lee BB, Kim DI, Huh S, et al. New experiences with absolute ethanol sclerotherapy in the management of a complex form of congenital venous malformation. *J Vasc Surg*. 2001.

51. Lee BB, Do YS, Byun HS, et al. Advanced management of venous malformation with ethanol sclerotherapy: mid-term results. *J Vasc Surg.* 2003;37:533–538.

52. Mattassi R. Differential diagnosis in congenital vascular-bone syndromes. *Semin Vasc Surg.* 1993.

53. Belov ST. Correction of lower limbs length discrepancy in congenital vascular-bone disease by vascular surgery performed during childhood. *Semin Vasc Surg.* 1993.

54. Ziyeh S, Spreer J, Rossler J, et al. Parkes Weber or Klippel-Trenaunay syndrome? Non-invasive diagnosis with MR projection angiography. *Eur Radiol.* 2004.

55. Szuba A, Skobe M, Karkkainen MJ, et al. Therapeutic lymphangiogenesis with human recombinant VEGF-C. *FASEB J.* 2002;16:1985–1987.

56. Bridenbaugh E. Literature watch. *Lymphat Res Biol.* 2005.

5
Medical Management of Lymphedema

Cheryl L. Morgan

Historical Review

While chapter 1 documents the early lymphatic discoveries, many of today's interventions developed from investigations into the causes and management of lymphedema over the past 2 centuries.

In the 1870s, Still, the founder of the American School of Osteopathy, created an approach to manual therapies acknowledging the lymphatics as a vital system and designed to correct anatomical deviations that interfered with the flow of lymph and blood. Still proposed a relationship in which cerebrospinal fluid is reabsorbed by the lymph, a relationship supported by recent research (1).

In the 1890s, Winiwarter, an Austrian physician from Vienna, described a treatment for swollen limbs that seems surprisingly similar to that recommended today; the conservative treatment included elevation, compression, massage, and exercise. Unfortunately, Winiwarter's suggestions were not advanced further for some time (2).

A few decades later, in the 1920s, Miller developed the Miller thoracic pump technique, which he described as effective in creating intrathoracic pressure changes on lymphatic flow. Many of the conditions that he treated successfully with this technique include forms of edema (3,4).

In 1922, Millard published the first osteopathic medical textbook examining only the lymphatic system, *Applied Anatomy of the Lymphatics*, and was the founder and president of the International Lymphatic Research Society in Kirksville, MO (5).

In the 1930s, Vodder and his wife began working with manual techniques to affect lymph flow.

Although the Vodders were Danish, the majority of their work was performed and published in France, where they lived and worked from 1928 to 1939. Here they developed their technique, then called lymph drainage massage. They later coined the term manual lymph drainage. The Vodder technique of lymph drainage is the most widely taught component of conservative lymphedema treatment (6,7).

In the 1960s, Asdonk, a German physician, scientifically tested the Vodder technique of manual lymph drainage in his clinic on 20 000 patients. From this research, he established the indications, contraindications, and effects of the techniques (8).

In the following decade, the Földis combined the Vodders' manual lymph drainage with bandaging, exercise, and specific skin care into the treatment program termed complete decongestive physiotherapy (CDP), later renamed complete decongestive therapy (CDT) (9). The Földis' many contributions to lymphology include their extensive research as well as directing the Földi Clinic in Germany.

The first North American lymphedema treatment centers opened in the 1980s, where specially trained therapists initiate the use of CDT to treat lymphedema patients.

In the 1990s, an increase of scientific literature, patient awareness, and interested therapists and physicians stimulates an increase of treatment centers in the United States. In 1992, Medicare (KS) approves CDT treatment for lymphedema. In 1999, a new CPT code describing manual therapies, including manual lymph drainage (97140), is approved by the American Medical Association.

In recent years, continued use of CDT has encouraged controlled clinical studies and research to focus on quality of life, treatment outcomes, and cost effectiveness. The American Society of Lymphology (ASL) has initiated efforts to standardize educational requirements of health care professionals treating disorders of the lymphatics. Legislation has been introduced by the National Lymphedema Network (NLN) to improve reimbursement for medical supplies for lymphedema. Research has moved to the forefront thanks to the Lymphatic Research Foundation (LRF).

Among individuals, Australian physicians Casley-Smith devoted more than 40 years to research, treatment, and the education of therapists (10). Their abundant and diverse research using the electron microscope has received worldwide recognition.

The significant contributions through the Centers for Disease Control and Prevention led by Dreyer and Addiss in the treatment of filarial lymphedema and vector control (11) have produced extraordinary developments that will benefit millions suffering with disfiguring consequences of parasitic infection.

Witte, a professor and general surgeon, made major contributions as a researcher and educator (12). He and his wife, also a professor of surgery, established the first lymphological laboratory in the United States devoted to both basic and clinical investigation of lymphatic circulatory disorders.

Many of these accomplishments above could not have been realized without the contributions of medical professionals, such as the prominent physicians Guyton and Stemmer (13,14). The prolific research of Olzsewski and Partsch continue to contribute to the develop of treatment options and new diagnostic methods to improve equally the quality of research, medical intervention, and the quality of life of lymphedema patients.

Successful Treatment for Lymphedema

Optimal treatment results require patient adherence. This begins with an accurate diagnosis, as outlined in chapter 2. To date, complete deconges-

tive therapy is recognized internationally as the most successful treatment option for lymphedema (15,16). Other names used to describe the program include complete (or combined, or complex) decongestive physiotherapy (17).

The author has designated the term Comprehensive Decongestive Therapy©, to indicate that therapeutic interventions may not have complete results, and need not be considered complex. This program, introduced in 1989, also includes comprehensive instruction in the disease, its treatment, and the expected results. Nutritional counseling and psychosocial intervention, e.g. counseling, support groups, and resource management, are essential components of the program as well. These additional components are described on pages 51 and 52. The results of this program are demonstrated by one patient's progress through treatment (see Figures 5-1 to 5-8).

A fundamental CDT-based program described by the International Society of Lymphology includes manual lymph drainage, specialized

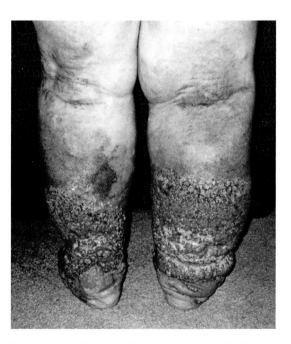

FIGURE 5-1. A 51-year-old female presenting with bilateral, chronic, stage III lymphedema (elephantiasis). Vena cava clipping 25 years prior following orthopedic surgery and deep vein thrombosis was performed to prevent reoccurring pulmonary embolism. Massive lymphedema developed despite the patient's efforts to obtain medical intervention. (Photo courtesy of CL Morgan.)

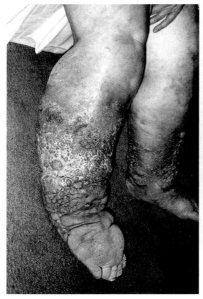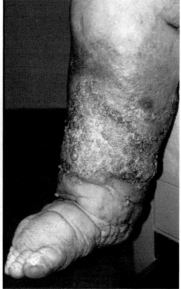

A

B

FIGURE 5-2. (A) Allergies prevent antibiotic therapy to control infection. Ulcerations have persisted for 17 years. Patient is unable to ambulate, exercise, or stand without extreme discomfort. (B) Venous studies revealed complete venous incompetence of deep venous system. Large superficial varicose veins provide collateral flow over lower trunk. (Photos courtesy of CL Morgan.)

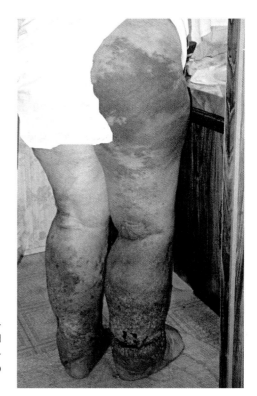

FIGURE 5-3. Recurrent episodes of infection complicated progress. Laboratory tests revealed numerous bacterial and fungal infections that continued to occur during the first 10 weeks of treatment. During these periods, compression was discontinued and the volume of edema increased. (Photo courtesy of CL Morgan.)

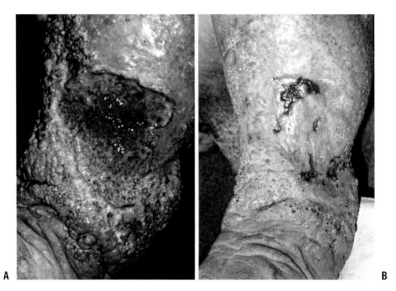

A **B**

FIGURE 5-4. (A) A Stage IV ulceration measured 28.4 cm by 14.3 cm. Treatment was initiated with bedrest, elevation of the lower extremity, and compression-aided wound care. Dressing changes were required hourly. Surface infections were treated with a 2% benzethonium chloride solution, and the ulcer base debrided with trypsin gel. Manual lymph drainage and passive range of motion were initiated at the second week, once wound drainage was reduced and episodes of infection were under control. (B) Here fibrosclerotic tissues have begun to soften, hyperpigmentation has improved, episodes of infection have been reduced, and ulcers have decreased in diameter. Wounds are treated daily with non-ionic isotonic surfactant cleanser and polymeric membrane dressing once infections have resolved. Dressing changes are required every 2 to 3 hours. (Photos courtesy of CL Morgan.)

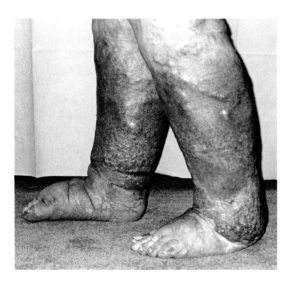

FIGURE 5-5. At 33 weeks, the wounds have closed without surgical intervention. Papillomas have been excised, and are benign. There is no episode of infection for 8 weeks. Patient is able to ambulate, stand, increase exercise, donn and doff bandages following instruction in self-care program. (Photograph courtesy of CL Morgan.)

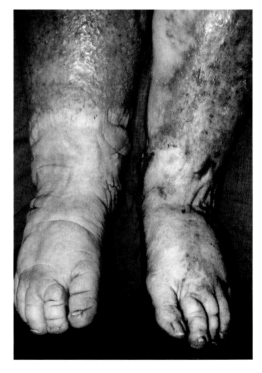

FIGURE 5-6. Results of comprehensive treatment after 47 weeks. No recurrence of wounds. Bilateral bandaging is applied by the patient each evening. The patient has returned to work. Circumference of the lower limbs has been reduced and continued improvement is expected with demonstrated adherence to a self-care program. (Photo courtesy of CL Morgan and LL Tretbar.)

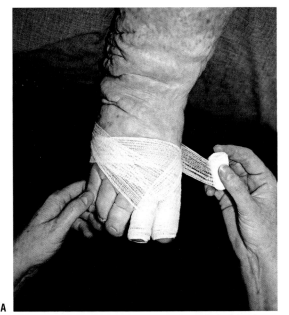

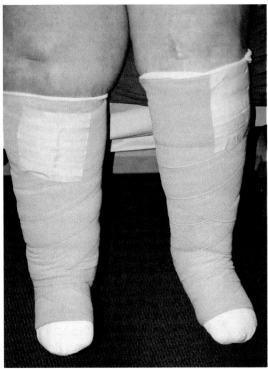

A

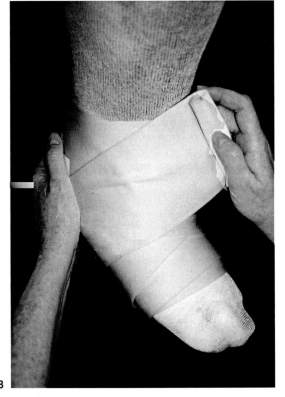

B

FIGURE 5-8. The patient has returned to all normal activities and has continued with intermittent week-long treatment sessions twice per year to improve the integrity of tissue and improve bandaging techniques as progress continues. Results have been sustained, without recurrent ulceration or a decrease in functional abilities achieved during the initial course of treatment 14 years ago. (Photo courtesy of CL Morgan and LL Tretbar.)

FIGURE 5-7. (A) Review of bandaging techniques performed with patient improves patient adherence and self care skills. (B) An example of bandaging used for lymphedema management taught to the patient for intensive program and subsequent self-care. The patient is now able to wear shoes and increase activity.

bandaging, exercise, skin care, and a self-management program (16).

The goals of intervention are to improve the integrity of the affected skin and connective tissues, to reduce or eliminate infections, to reduce edema, and to facilitate patients' ability to manage their condition once the intensive treatment phase is completed.

Two-Phase Intervention

The management of lymphedema using CDT is divided into 2 phases. The first addresses the primary need of the patient, such as treatment of the swollen limb, increased functional capacity, and prevent infections. Trained health care professionals initiate the first phase with CDT. The second phase addresses the continuing needs of the patient through self-management.

Many European models of CDT recommend twice daily treatment visits for an average of 4 to 6 weeks. However, constraints of insurance carriers limit this successful model and, subsequently, the results. Patients with upper extremity lymphedema might receive daily treatments for 3 to 4 weeks, whereas those with lower extremity lymphedema might receive an average of 4 to 6 weeks of daily visits. Some clinics report that patients may receive CDT only 1 to 3 times per week, due to insurance limitations, work limitations, or physical distances traveled.

Health professionals must be aware that symptom reversal is a slow process. Even in the best circumstances where appropriate intervention occurs and patient adherence is optimal, symptom reversal may require 8 months or more of treatment. When improper treatment or rapidly paced shortcuts are employed, patients rarely have lasting outcomes and often experience exacerbation of their symptoms. Frequently, individuals with comorbidities do not respond as quickly to treatment.

The components of the 2-phase treatment method are:

Phase I: Intensive Treatment

- manual lymph drainage
- skin care (including wound care if indicated)
- bandaging (specialized)
- exercise (in bandages)
- compression garment (if appropriate)

Phase II: Self-management

- skin care
- manual lymphatic drainage (as needed)
- daytime compression garment, nighttime bandaging
- exercise (in bandages or garment)
- support groups

Manual Lymph Drainage

Manual lymph drainage is based on physiologic principles that regulate the flow of lymph, and it influences the general lymph circulation primar-

ily by affecting the initial and superficial lymphatics. The techniques are designed to stimulate lymph flow from distal lymphatics to proximal lymphatics (7,18). This objective requires that manual lymph drainage move excess lymph from the swollen areas or sites of obstruction, to adjacent areas that can efficiently transport the additional volume.

To facilitate lymph flow into adjacent body areas, manual techniques include treatment of the contralateral or ipsilateral lymph node regions. Lymphography and lymphoscintigraphy, used for research and diagnostic purposes, confirm that superficial lymph fluid moves around blocked areas toward more central vessels when these specialized manual techniques are used (15,16).

Manual lymph drainage has many effects on the lymph system by:

- increasing lymph transport capacity, thereby increasing the volume of lymph fluid transported proximally
- increasing the frequency of lymph vessel contractions
- increasing pressure in the lymph collector vessels
- redirecting natural flow patterns toward collateral vessels, anastomoses, and uninvolved lymph node regions
- increasing arteriolar blood flow

A concept, now under investigation, suggests that manual lymph drainage enhances angiogenesis; if true, the number of functioning lymphatics should increase. Another theory under investigation is that the compression bandages are responsible for the promotion of angiogenesis.

Starting Manual Lymph Drainage

Before initiating treatment, the program should be reviewed with the patient by the referring physician and therapist. Physician support greatly increases patient adherence to an intensive therapy program. The physician should know that mobilizing the lymphatic fluid will cause a temporary increase in circulating blood volume. Confirm with the physician if there are any comorbidities that would contraindicate CDT (see Summary at end of Chapter, page 53). Once these issues are settled, treatment may begin (19).

Manual lymph drainage recruits functioning lymph vessels and nodes closest to the regions that are not adequately performing. Therefore, regardless of the site of insufficient flow, treatment can include manual work on the neck, back, abdominal region, and uninvolved inguinal and axillary lymph nodes (6,16,18). Initially, manual therapy begins from the contralateral trunk area toward the congested area. Treatment then continues to move from the involved area to uninvolved areas.

The manual techniques of manual lymph drainage are light, slow, and precise. Manual lymph drainage does not use the deep strokes and pressures of effleurage, a standard therapeutic massage technique. Rather, a specified number of light pressure strokes without friction that directionally stretch tissue are used (6,18,20,21). The manual lymph drainage therapy session usually requires a minimum of 45 to 60 minutes, depending on the size of the limb(s) or body parts involved, the severity of the symptoms, and the amount of fibrosis (20).

Skin Care

Meticulous skin care is an essential component of both treatment phases. The goal of careful and thorough skin care is to avoid or eliminate fungal and bacterial infections such as cutaneous cellulitis, erysipelas, or lymphangitis (22). Patients with lymphedema experience skin changes and are highly susceptible to infections. Dermatological conditions often associated with lymphedema can include:

- dry skin
- hyperkeratosis
- contact dermatitis
- lipodermatosclerosis
- fungal infections
- folliculitis
- lymph fistulas
- papillomatosis
- lymphangiectasia
- lymphorrhea
- eczema

- dermatolymphangioadenitis (DLA) (cellulitis, lymphangitis, erysipelas)
- lymphangiosarcoma
- chronic ulceration

The protein-rich fluid that accumulates in the lymphedematous tissues serves as a culture medium for pathogens which circulate within the body or enter through skin lesions (23,24).

Wound Care

When the integrity of the skin is compromised by chronic edema or lymphedema, regardless of the etiology, basic skin care regimens can reduce the risk of complications from small lesions to chronic ulcers (23,24). Should a wound develop with lymphedema, compression-aided wound care methods are critical for the patient's continued progress (25).

Bandaging

Because skin elasticity is partially lost in lymphedema, tissue hydrostatic pressures must be maintained by the use of external support. This support must be continuous until the volume reduction stabilizes and tissues remodel with improved functional lymphatic capacity (25).

During the treatment phase, bandaging performed by a health care professional with specialized training will achieve the best results. A specific combination of padding, foam, protective gauze, and short-stretch bandages is applied in precise layers following each session of manual lymph drainage. Before lymphedema bandaging, the involved skin is cleansed and protected with an appropriate moisturizer; in the case of ulcerations, protective dressing that sufficiently captures exudate is applied. Experienced lymphologists recognize that most of the success observed during the treatment phase is due to compression bandaging (2,23,25,26).

Bandaging affects the entire lymphatic system by:

- providing support for tissues that have lost elasticity
- improving muscle pump efficiency during activity

- reducing the rate of ultrafiltration
- facilitating colloidal protein reabsorption
- softening fibrotic tissue with localized pressure
- providing a mild increase in tissue pressure, assisting lymph vessels to empty
- reducing the hydrostatic pressure gradient between blood and lymphatic tissues, thus preventing refilling of the interstitium with fluid

Types of Bandages

A distinction must be made between short-stretch (low elastic) bandages and long-stretch (high elastic) bandages and the type of compression that each offers.

As their name implies, short-stretch bandages have little or no stretch in them. When applied to the limb, they form an envelope or cocoon around the limb. In the resting state, compression is minimal but constant. Compression develops only during exercise as the muscles expand and press against the wrap. Therefore, exercise is important for the effect of short-stretch bandages to be optimized. Because of the low resting pressure, they can be worn at night (25–27).

Long-stretch bandages are highly elastic and allow extension to perhaps 3 times their resting length. Thus they create a continuous compression on the limb with a high resting pressure. However, during exercise they stretch as the muscles expand and the compressive force decreases. This diminution of force follows the Laplace law ($P = T/r$) that states that external pressure (P) is directionally proportional to the tension (T) of the elastic fabric, and inversely proportional to the radius (r) (25). Because of high resting pressure, these bandages are not recommended for wear at night; the pressure can compromise arterial circulation and already compromised tissues, especially over bony prominences (25,27).

Although bandages can be cumbersome patients should continue, if not increase, their activity level to facilitate muscle pumps and stimulate lymphatic function. After a period of adjustment, most bandages are well tolerated by informed and motivated patients. For optimum patient adherence, patients should thoroughly understand the importance of the bandages during the treatment phase. During this period the bandages are worn continuously except for the time required to cleanse, treat, or rewrap the limb. Patients and their families

often begin to learn to apply the bandage toward the middle of the treatment phase (16,20,23).

The bandaging portion of a treatment session may require 20 to 90 minutes; the amount of time depends on the number of custom foam pieces to be produced, how much patient education and assistance is required, how many limbs are affected, the size of the involved limb(s) or body parts, and if any lesions require care.

By the third or fourth week of the treatment phase, the clinician will spend less time actively bandaging, concentrating on instructing the patient in basic application and technique. The patient's progress may yet require alterations in custom pieces, education, and modifications in application to continue improvement. Patient education is necessary to safely and accurately apply lymphedema bandages. Regular monitoring by a qualified health care professional is essential and highly recommended.

Exercise

During the intensive treatment phase, exercises are performed while wearing lymphedema bandages. The exercise program, customized to a patient's functional ability, includes activities that promote the emptying of the affected lymph regions. The activities should also assist the functioning lymphatics to work more efficiently. During the self-management phase, when the patient has achieved a reasonable volume reduction, a compression garment may be worn (23,27).

The amount of time spent on exercise during a session in the treatment phase will vary, based on the number of measured limitations and the intervention goals. Strategies for conserving energy and achieving balance between exercise and rest should be developed for each person. If there are no other existing functional limitations, a patient may be able to accept responsibility for exercise even during the initial treatment phase (28,29).

Many patients with lymphedema experience some level of limitation in joint range of motion, muscle strength, and posture or gait deficits. Any such limitations should be considered when developing an exercise program for the patient.

Exercise improves cardiovascular function, muscular strength, functional capacity, and endurance (28). Combinations of resistance, aerobic, and flexibility programs may be beneficial in controlling lymphedema and assist those patients with mobility or joint function limitations. The topic of exercise is still controversial. Therefore, current information should be presented to patients to assist them in making decisions about the most beneficial activities.

Compression Garments

Near the end of the intensive treatment phase, if the compromised limb or body part has reached normal or near normal size, a compression garment may be selected to enable to patient to better manage a self-care program. In the earliest stage of lymphedema or for those at risk of developing lymphedema, compression garments may be appropriate intervention (29). The elastic support garments are worn during the day to prevent reaccumulation of fluid. Many patients continue with bandaging for a period of time during the self-management phase to enhance the results achieved (30).

Compression garments affect the lymph system by:

- maintaining hydrostatic pressure that prevents refilling of the interstitial space with lymph fluid
- preserving long-term reductions of limb circumference achieved by CDT
- continue the softening of fibrotic tissues initiated during the treatment phase

Compression Garment Selection

An experienced and trained compression specialist with a thorough understanding of lymphedema, is best qualified to make the detailed decisions of garment selection, e.g. the appropriate pressure gradient and correct style and fit. Many patients report reversal of progress or complications when using a garment that is poorly fit.

Results from the intensive treatment (Phase I) and self-management (Phase II) are jeopardized without the use of some form of compression, avoiding the use of garments until optimal or near normal limb reduction has been reached. Well-informed patients understand that compression is

essential for sustained results of lymphedema management (27). There are numerous garment manufacturers, designs, and options now available to compression therapy specialists. Many lymphedema therapists are well trained in fitting several products and are better suited to assist patients with these choices.

Compression Pumps

Another form of compression is the pneumatic pump. Internationally, there is considerable debate over the effectiveness of these devices. Providing intermittent (IPC) or sequential (SCD) compression, these devices are thought to reduce edema by decreasing capillary filtration. They can be effective in venous insufficiency, dependent edemas, lymphovenous stasis, and in palliative care (31).

The interventions above are the components of CDT described by the International Society of Lymphology.

Comprehensive Approach

The authors' program, Comprehensive Decongestive Therapy ©, includes the following additional components of care: nutritional counseling, psychosocial intervention, and patient instruction.

Nutritional Counseling

Whether a patient is faced with complications of nutritional deficits from chronic illness, wounds, obesity, diabetes, or the effects of chemotherapy, nutritional status must be considered during the treatment program. The frequent coexistence of lymphedema and obesity suggests that obesity may contribute to the development of lymphedema in some cases (32). Laboratory work collected at the start of therapy or 30 days prior is a valuable clinical evaluation tool and is effective in developing a comprehensive plan of care that will optimize the patients' results and strengthen the lifestyle changes necessary for lifelong management (33,34).

Coordinating nutritional recommendations with the patient's physician(s) is paramount for a successful program. A registered dietician or clinical nutritionist can provide this service.

Psychosocial Intervention

An integral part of this approach is the provision of support for patients and their family or caregivers to take a positive role in daily management of their condition(s). Encouraging participation in the process and results (adherence) is preferential to compliance (35). Some patients with advanced disease require palliative care and a well-organized clinical team to address the physical and psychological needs presented. Many patients with lymphedema have concomitant health concerns, which contribute to psychosocial problems such as depression, isolation, loneliness, anxiety, and poor coping skills (36,37).

Initial assessment of a patient's quality of life, the need for community resources (e.g. transportation, financial assistance, supplies), and individual counseling or support groups promotes increased adherence to the intensive phase of therapy (32,38). Another successful therapeutic tool for recovery and coping with chronic illness is art therapy (39,40). These services can be provided by a professional therapist or counselor, a licensed clinical social worker, or a psychologist.

Patient Instruction

The establishment of a comprehensive program requires a structured and thorough patient education component that can be individualized. Education about the condition, effective treatment and results, instruction in problem solving, nutritional guidelines, programs for exercise, and information on proper hygiene, skin care, and care of bandages and garments all provide a foundation for improved adherence and outcomes of therapy (41). All members of the clinical team provide this service.

Phase II, Self-management

Some patients or their caregivers are candidates for training in some of the manual techniques to assist in self-management. They must be carefully instructed and educated in the appropriate pressures and directions of the strokes to avoid exacerbation of the symptoms. If a patient experiences an increase in swelling or a plateau in reduction following the treatment phase, follow-up with additional sessions of manual lymph drainage in the clinic is appropriate. A patient who reports increased swelling should be examined and cleared of possible complications, such as recurrent malignancy, before continuing treatment. At this point, manual therapy may enhance the gains achieved during the initial treatment phase. Once the intensive treatment phase is complete, most patients have learned how to manage their condition with bandaging. The progress achieved and severity or persistence of the symptoms determine whether a patient continues to wear bandages at night. Most patients apply the bandages at night to optimize improvements in tissue integrity and volume reduction during the self-management phase.

Patients often report that their symptoms fluctuate with climate, body weight, and changes in lifestyle. Most concur that lymphedema is best managed with consistent use of all components of the self-management phase. During the self-management phase, patients wear the compression garments during daytime hours and continue with bandaging at night. As a result of the education provided during the intensive treatment (Phase 1), the patient should understand and be able to perform donning, doffing, and care of both bandages and compression garments.

Many patients will need to wear a compression garment for the remainder of their lives to effectively control symptoms and retain reduction of volume achieved. Nevertheless, tissue swelling and fibrosis can occur in nearby areas if garments fit poorly. Patients must remain attentive to any tissue changes in involved or adjacent areas. Garment fit and condition should be checked at least every 6 months, particularly if the patient experiences difficulties with fit, comfort, or symptom control.

Patients are encouraged to continue their exercise program while wearing compression during the self-management phase. Periodic clinic visits may be needed to review the self-management home program or to modify for improvements or decline in function (42).

Summary

Complex decongestive therapy has proven to be an effective treatment protocol for lymphedema management for more than 70 years (23,27,42). It cannot be overly emphasized that it is essential for health professionals to obtain in-depth education about lymphedema and related disorders and specialized training in each of the therapeutic interventions. Of equal importance is that they acquire extensive experience to adequately prepare for designation as a lymphedema specialist.

Additional indications for CDT include the following:

- chronic venous insufficiency
- post-thrombotic (deep venous thrombosis) syndrome
- chronic wounds (associated with edema)
- traumatic edema (iatrogenic, postsurgical, post-musculoskeletal injury)
- complex regional pain syndrome (CRPS), formerly known as reflex sympathetic dystrophy
- rheumatoid arthritis
- possibly lipedema

There are some contraindications or precautions to CDT/manual lymph drainage to be noted. Most patients will tolerate the treatment, since it is a gentle, smooth manual approach rather than a deep powerful massage. However, monitoring of cardiac, pulmonary, and renal functions is still necessary because of the temporary increase of blood volume. The following are relative contraindications and precautions to CDT:

- acute infections, local or systemic, viral or bacterial: cellulitis, erysipelas
- secondary acute inflammation
- acute bronchitis or bronchial asthma (uncontrolled)
- diabetes
- cardiac failure, hypertension
- malignancy
- renal insufficiency
- sclerotic arteries or venous insufficiency (in patients above age 60 years)
- hyperthyroidism or hypothyroidism
- pregnancy
- recent surgery
- Crohn disease, diverticulitis
- deep venous thrombosis, acute superficial thrombophlebitis

References

1. Still AT. *The Philosophy and Mechanical Principles of Osteopathy*. Kansas City, MO: Hudson-Kimberly; 1902;65–66.
2. Földi M, Kubik S, eds. *Lehrbuch der Lymphologie für Mediziner*. 5th ed. Munich-Jena: Urban & Fisher; 2002.
3. Miller CE. The mechanics of lymphatic circulation. *J Am Osteopath Assoc*. 1923;22:397–398.
4. Miller CE. Osteopathic principles and thoracic pump therapeutics proved by scientific research. *J Am Osteopath Assoc*. 1927;26:910–914.
5. Millard FP. *Applied Anatomy of the Lymphatics*. Kirksville, MO: AG Walmstey ed. International Lymphatic Research Society; 1922.
6. Vodder E. *Le drainage lymphatique, une nouvelle méthode thérapeutique*. Santé Pour Tous: Paris, 1936.
7. Wittlinger H, Wittlinger G. *Introduction to Dr. Vodder's Manual Lymph Drainage*. Heidelberg: Haug; 1986.
8. Asdonk J. *Lymphdrainage und Molekularmassage. Phys Medizin und Rehabilitation, Heft*. 1967;10: 62–65.
9. Földi E, Földi M, Weissleder H. Conservative treatment of lymphedema of the limbs. *Angiology*. 1985;36:171–180.
10. Casley-Smith JR. *The Pathophysiology of Lymphoedema*. In: Heim LR, ed. IXth International Society of Lymphology. Tel Ariv, Israel. Immunology Research Foundation, Newburgh, USA, 1983:125–130.
11. Dreyer G, Addiss D, Dreyer P, et al. *Basic Lymphoedema Management, Treatment and Prevention of Problems Associated with Lymphatic Filariasis*. Hollis, NH: Hollis Publishing; 2002.
12. Bernas MJ, Witte CL, Witte MH. The diagnosis and treatment of peripheral lymphedema. *Lymphology*. 2001;34:84–91.
13. Guyton AC, Granger HJ, Taylor AE. Interstitial fluid pressures. *Physiol Rev*. 1971;51:527–563.
14. Stemmer R. Ein klinisches Zeichen zur Früh-und Differentialdiagnose des Lymphodems. *Vasa*. 1976;5(3):261–262.
15. Browse N, Burnand K, Mortimer P, eds. *Diseases of the Lymphatics*. London: Arnold; 2003.
16. Weissleder H, Schuchhardt C, eds. *Lymphedema: Diagnosis and Therapy*. Bonn: Kagerer Kommunikation; 1997.
17. International Society of Lymphology. The diagnosis and treatment of peripheral lymphedema. Consensus Document of the International Society of Lymphology. *Lymphology*. 2003;36:84–91.
18. Kasseroller RG. *Compendium of Dr. Vodder's Manual Lymph Drainage*. Heidelberg: Haug; 1998.
19. Browse NL, Stewart G. Lymphoedema: pathophysiology and classification. *J Cardiovasc Surg*. Torino, 1985;26:156–168.
20. Mortimer PS. Managing lymphedema. *Clin Exp Dermatol*. 1995;20:98–106.

21. Eliska O, Eliskova M. Are peripheral lymphatics damaged by high-pressure manual massage? *Lymphology*. 1995;28:21–30.

22. Olszewski WL. *Lymph Stasis: Pathophysiology, Diagnosis and Treatment*. Boston: CRC Press; 1991.

23. Weissleder H, Schuchhardt C, eds. *Lymphedema: Diagnosis and Therapy*. 3rd ed. Bonn: Kagerer Kommunikation; 2001.

24. Olszewski WL, Jamal S. Recurrent dermatolymphangioadenitis (DLA) is responsible for progression of lymphedema. Progress in Lymphology XV. *Lymphology*. 1996;(Suppl.)29:331–334.

25. Partsch H, Rabe E, Stemmer R. *Compression Therapy of the Extremities*. Paris: Editions Phlébologiques; 2000.

26. Partsch H. Understanding the pathophysiological effects of compression. In: *European Wound Management Association*. Position Document. Understanding compression therapy. London: MEP Ltd.; 2003;2–4.

27. Földi E, Földi E, Weissleder H. Conservative treatment of lymphedema of the limbs. *Anbiology* 1985;36:171–180.

28. Casley-Smith, JR, Mason MR, et al. Complex physical therapy for the lymphedematous leg. *Int J Angio*. 1995;4:134–142.

29. Pappas CJ, O'Donnell TF, Kalisher L, et al. Long-term results of compression treatment of lymphedema. *J Vasc Surg*. 1992;16(4):555–564.

30. Badger CMA, Peacock JL, Mortimer PS. A randomized controlled, parallel-group clinical trial comparing multi-layer bandaging with hosiery versus hosiery alone in the treatment of lymphedema of the limb. *Cancer*. 2000;88(12):2832–2837.

31. Vowden K. The use of intermittent pneumatic compression in venous ulceration. *Br J Nurs*. 2001;10(8):491–509.

32. Mortimer PS. The pathophysiology of lymphedema. *Cancer*. 1998;(Am Suppl.)12(83):2798–2802.

33. Olszewski WL, Engeset A. Immune proteins, enzymes, and electrolytes in human peripheral lymph. *Lymphology*. 1978;11:156.

34. Ryan TJ, Mallon EC. Lymphatics and the processing of antigen, *Clin Dermatol*. 1995;13(5):485–492.

35. McWayne J, Heiney SP. Psychologic and social sequelae of secondary lymphedema: a review. *Cancer*. 2005;104:457–466.

36. Azevedo WF, Boccardo F, Zilli A, et al. A reliable and valid quality of life in patients with lymphedema—version of the SF-36. *Lymphology*. 2002;35(1):177–180.

37. De Godoy JMP, Braile DM, et al. Quality of life and peripheral lymphedema. *Lymphology*. 2002;35(2):44–45.

38. Falvo D. Medical and psychosocial aspects of chronic illness and disability. Jones and Bartlettt, Sudbury, MA, 2005.

39. Rubin JA. *Art as Therapy*. Psychology Press: 1999.

40. Malchiodi CA. *Handbook of Art Therapy*. Guilford Press. 2003.

41. Hwang JH, Kwon JY, Lee BB, et al. Changes in lymphatic function after complex physical therapy for lymphedema. *Lymphology*. 1999;32(1):15–21.

42. Lee BB. Chronic lymphedema, no more stepchild to modern medicine. *Eur J Lymphology*. 2004;14:6–12.

6
Surgical Management of Lymphedema

B.B. Lee
With contributions from V. Krylov and C. Becker

Introduction

An ideal treatment for the lymphedematous limb should restore both function and cosmetic appearance. Unfortunately, it is impossible to achieve these goals using current treatment modalities.

Although manual lymph drainage-based complete decongestive therapy (CDT) effectively controls the progression of the disease in most cases and remains the primary management for chronic lymphedema, surgical therapy provides an adjunct to nonsurgical treatments (1–8).

Surgical treatments of lymphedema are usually categorized as excisional (ablative) or reconstructive (9–28). As with all forms of lymphedema treatment, surgical management necessitates a lifetime commitment to treatment. It too has limitations similar to those of conservative treatment, e.g. failure to improve the lymphedematous limb and the inability to prevent progression of the disease (29,30). Surgical treatment, whether ablative or reconstructive, has many advocates and is known to provide control of chronic lymphedema. Reconstructive surgery, in particular, has an attractive theoretical basis that in the future might provide an opportunity for cure. The use of reconstructive surgery, however, remains controversial and unavailable to most clinicians.

A dedicated and experienced microsurgical team for lymphovenous and lympholymphatic anastomoses is a prerequisite for successful long-term results (15,17,19,21,23). Unfortunately, only a limited number of institutions have surgical teams that can meet these conditions.

As stated previously, CDT must accompany any type of surgical treatment, the combination of which may achieve complementary benefits not obtained by CDT alone (31,32).

Excisional/Ablative Surgery

Excisional procedures, often known as reduction or debulking operations, remove scarred and disfigured lymphedematous tissue from the limb. These procedures were condemned for many years because of general morbidity and significant complications; their application had been nonselective and used for any type of lymphedema. Some of these once-abandoned operations, however, have been reassessed and provide alternative palliative operations for chronic end-stage lymphedema. Large numbers of long-term results have yet to be assessed.

Early Debulking Operations

Excisional procedures have been described by Charles in 1912, Sistrunk in 1918, Homans in 1936, and Thompson in 1962 (9,10,12,13,33).

Charles recommended a radical operation for reducing the size of a massively swollen calf or foot (33). The entire skin and subcutaneous fat of the lower leg are removed circumferentially to the muscular fascia. Split-thickness skin grafts are applied over the denuded areas. The excision includes major veins and nerves of the saphenous system in addition to the lymphedematous tissues. The foot can be selectively treated in a similar manner.

Sistrunk described a noncircumferential debulking procedure. It removes a wedge of skin and subcutaneous fat to the muscular fascia (12). Skin grafting is not required inasmuch as the adjacent flaps, created by the excision, are approximated and sutured.

Homans extended Sistrunk's operation (10). He first excised a medial wedge of lymphedematous calf tissue then undermined the flaps to extend the area of tissue removal. Today, these 2 surgical approaches may be combined to reduce the circumference of the thigh.

Thompson's operation is seldom performed today because it failed to provide relief of symptoms. Its thesis suggested that the lymphatics of transected skin (dermis), if buried beneath the deep muscular fascia, would form a bridge between the 2 lymph systems. The anticipated drainage from superficial to deep lymphatics failed to develop (12,13).

Selection of Candidates for Excisional Surgery

Failure to obtain satisfactory control of the lymphedematous process or to prevent disease progression during a year of vigorous nonsurgical treatment is a major criterion for selection for surgical treatment (29,32). Another important criterion, for any type of lymphatic surgery, is a serious commitment to a lifetime of maintenance. Because postoperative maintenance care with CDT relies heavily on a self-initiated, home-based maintenance program, it requires an initial hospital-based educational program for both patient and family (32).

A multidisciplinary team should evaluate all candidates for surgery. The final selection should be made by consensus after a vigorous and critical assessment is performed. Patients with lymphedema in clinical stage IV or those progressing to stage III with profound soft tissue changes, hardened fibrosclerotic tissues with distortion, disfigurement, and/or elephantiasis are ideal candidates for excisional surgery. Sepsis should have recurred more than 3 times during the year, even under adequate antibiotic protection (31,32).

Surgery should be considered only when the epifascial (superficial) lymphatic system has been irreversibly damaged. As with all debulking operations, the surgical goal is to reduce the amount of fibrosclerotic lymphedematous tissue, to reduce the incidence of sepsis, and to improve the effectiveness of CDT.

Lymphoscintigraphy should demonstrate a progressive deterioration of the lymphatic system's residual function, e.g. increased dermal backflow, decreased lymph node uptake, decreased radiotracer clearance, and the disappearance of collaterals (34–36). Exclusion criteria include factors that interfere with conservative treatment and negate positive long-term results, such as poor compliance, lack of family support, age over 70 years, and infrequent infections.

Excisional Surgery

Our institution* uses a modified Auchincloss-Homans operation (9,10). It is usually performed on the lower limb and excises damaged skin and subcutaneous tissue to the muscular fascia. This procedure helps prevent tissue necrosis observed with procedures requiring more extensive undermining. Tissue edges are approximated and sutured immediately. As with many surgical procedures, morbidity consists of infection, hematoma, poor healing, skin loss, and recurrent swelling from lymphatic damage (11) (Figure 6-1).

Postoperatively, clinical evidence suggests increased lymph absorption through the deep subfascial lymphatic system, although lymphoscintigraphy has yet to confirm this clinical observation (29,32).

Liposuction

The swelling in a limb is often a combination of lymph fluid and edematous fat globules. It seems logical that removing at least 1 portion of the problem—the edematous fat—should improve the limb's condition.

Liposuction is a surgical technique that inserts a tiny cannula into the subcutaneous tissues and aspirates the surrounding fat (27,28). The imagined ease of performing liposuction (actually ablation by aspiration) created an intense inter-

---

*SamSung Medical Center & SungKyunKwan University, Seoul, Korea.

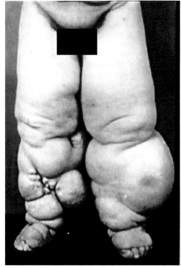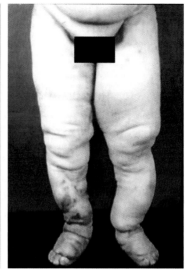

A   B

FIGURE 6-1. (A) Ablative (excisional) surgery might be considered when chronic lymphedema has reached end stage IV, as depicted here. These grossly disfigured legs create a problem in walking, hygiene, and social contact. Frequent infections and progressive lipodermatosclerosis have distorted the skin and subcutaneous structures. (B) Following excision of the fibroedematous tissue, an acceptable contour has been created. The patient now wears regular clothes and shoes and walks without a cane. Her response to CDT-based therapy has markedly improved, allowing her compression garments to be more easily fitted.

est within the surgical world when introduced in the 1980s. However, surgeons found that the procedure and its results were not always as satisfactory as hoped.

Treatment results of the arm with liposuction have been far better than those of the leg (28). A number of reasons have been given to explain the difference in results. The arm contains a greater percentage of fat per volume of tissue, thus permitting a greater volume removal, and there is usually less fibrosis in the arm's subcutaneous tissues, so fat removal can be more complete. Unfortunately, the desire for an easy outcome has been moderated by differing long-term results.

Each reported study emphasizes the need for continued compression to maintain the reduction of fluid. Brorson, having performed extensive studies of liposuction, has shown that arms treated with liposuction have retained their reduction in size at 5 years (27,28).

Many objections continue to be voiced to the use of liposuction, including that it damages normal lymphatics, there is little fat to be removed, and CDT alone may give equally good results (37).

Lymphatic Reconstructive Surgery

Of the various approaches to reconstructive surgery of the lymphatic system, procedures known as bypass operations have maintained credibility in the surgical community (14–16, 19–26). Occluded lymph-collecting vessels are bypassed with lymphovenous anastomoses. Normal distal lymphatics are anastomosed to proximal veins whose valvular functions appear normal.

Lympholymphatic anastomoses use normal distal lymph vessels attached to normal proximal lymphatics. These techniques are ideal for relieving obstructive lymphopathies and restoring normal lymphatic function (with the theoretic possibility of cure).

It is difficult, however, to intervene at the most efficacious time during the lymphedematous process, i.e. before lymph-collecting vessels are permanently damaged by lymph stasis (29,32). If one expects to reverse the functional paralysis in proximal lymph channels, the transposition of lymph vessels with normal peristaltic function is essential. Before reconstructive surgery can be widely accepted, either as an independent or an adjunctive therapy, positive long-term results must be demonstrated.

Selection of Candidates for Anastomotic/Reconstructive Surgery

In view of the massive financial, medical, and surgical commitments for reconstructive surgery, the screening of candidates for lymphovenous (19,20) or lympholymphatic (15,16) anastomotic surgery must be stringent (32).

To be considered for surgery, candidates must meet at least 3 criteria:

- show substantial clinical progression of the disease, from stage I to stage II or from stage II to stage III, in spite of an adequate 12-month CDP treatment program
- demonstrate progressive lymph fluid accumulation, especially below the knee, by lymphoscintigrams that show dermal backflow
- show decreasing effectiveness of manual lymph drainage-based CDT, especially below the knee

Treatment failure should be documented at least twice within a 6-month interval during a 2-year period.

Preoperative Evaluation

Before reconstructive lymphovenous or lympholymphatic anastomotic surgery is contemplated, the anatomic and functional status of the proximal lymph nodes and lymph-collecting vessels must be adequately assessed. Determination of function is necessary to identify normal, unparalyzed vessels (29,32).

Response to manual lymph drainage can be an indirect indication of the vessels functional status. Lymphoscintigraphy should be included in the preoperative evaluation to confirm these evaluations; additional information may be required from duplex ultrasonography. The newly available ultrasonographic lymphangiography and magnetic resonance lymphangiography (both in the investigative stage) are sometimes required to more accurately identify malfunctioning lymph-

collecting systems; their findings help confirm or rule out paralyzed lymph vessels (32).

Lymphovenous Anastomotic Surgery

Lymphovenous reconstruction is ideal for treating secondary lymphedema, which develops after cancer surgery or radiation, by restoring a more normal lymphatic function (21,30). Here there is selective damage to proximal lymph nodes, while distal lymph-collecting vessels remain intact. However, primary congenital lymphedema, with dysplasia of lymph nodes, is best treated by free lymph node transplantation (17,18).

The technique of lymphovenous anastomosis requires a microscopic end-to-end or end-to-side anastomosis between healthy, well-functioning lymphatic vessels and healthy veins (23,24). At minimum, 3 to 4 lymph-collecting vessels are anastomosed to defunctionalized branches of the saphenous or adjacent veins in the lower limb (19,20,25,26).

The operation can be performed at the inguinal (19,20) or popliteal level (23,24). The classic inguinal approach is preferred during the early stages of lymphedema, when good long-term results can be expected, e.g. in stage I before the collecting vessels are irreversibly paralyzed. A popliteal anastomosis may be necessary if the disease has progressed to a clinical stage II or early stage III. Evidence of progressive damage and paralysis of lymph-collecting vessels at the inguinal level further recommends a popliteal anastomosis (Figure 6-2).

Lympholymphatic Anastomotic Surgery

Lympholymphatic anastomotic reconstruction uses similar surgical principles and procedures (15,16). It is theoretically superior to a lymphovenous anastomosis, because it avoids the possibility of blood regurgitating into the lymph vessel and clotting.

Free Lymph Node Transplantation

The free lymph node transplantation technique is based on the principle of the free-flap autotrans-

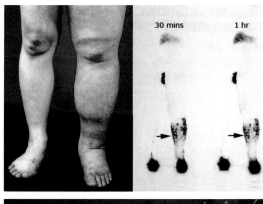

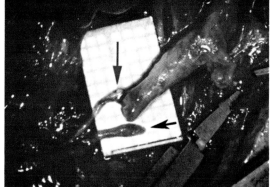

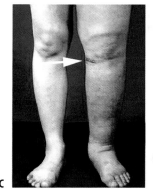

FIGURE 6-2. (A) Lymphovenous reconstructive surgery was performed on the left leg for progressive lymphedema, still in an early clinical stage. A preoperative lymphoscintigram shows marked dermal backflow (arrows). (B) This operative view of the popliteal area reveals functioning lymph-collecting vessels (arrows) that are to be anastomosed end-to-end to the defunctionalized vein above. (Russian method, modified by Krylov.) (C) One month after surgery, a good clinical response is noted, with less edema and improved skin turgor in the leg. The arrow points to the healing incision. A year later, dermal backflow is markedly diminished, as the scintigram demonstrates.

plantation technique (17,18). A vascularized pedicle flap is taken from the donor site, and a microscopic anastomosis is created between the flap and 1 or 2 sets of arteries and veins at the recipient site.

Lymphoscintigraphic evaluation is necessary to select the appropriate lymph node group for transplantation, e.g. inguinal, cervical, or axillary group (32). Adequate numbers of nodes must be left at the donor site, so that normal function can be maintained after harvesting. Selection of the best donor site is as important as selecting the best recipient site for transplantation. Otherwise, iatrogenic lymphedema may be induced by an unnecessarily aggressive nodal harvest. The patency and function of the patient's arterial and venous systems should be confirmed with ultrasonography as well. Local disease status at ankle, popliteal, or inguinal regions helps determine the recipient site.

The indications our institution adopted for free lymph node transplantation are more liberal than those for lymphovenous reconstructive surgery. The authors recommend free lymph node transplantation when lymphedema control is only minimal, or when there is suspicion of disease progression and increased sepsis (29,32) (Figure 6-3).

Vein Grafting

Another microsurgical technique uses free vein grafts to bridge lymphatic obstructions, either congenital or acquired. As with free nodal transplantation, long-term results are improved if the surgery is performed in the earlier stages of lymphedema. Campisi reported an 81% improvement, although the exact outcome criteria were not expressed (20).

Postoperative Management

After excisional or reconstructive surgery, continued CDT and compression are mandatory (32). When a successful free lymph node transplant is performed in stage II, CDT may be needed for 12 months or less (18). However, lymphovenous anastomotic surgery, performed for the

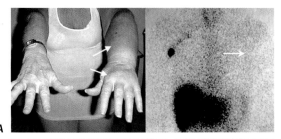

A

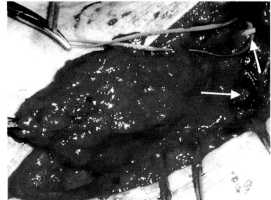

B

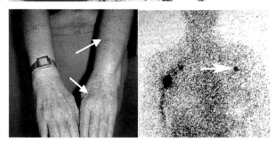

C

FIGURE 6-3. (A) Lymphedema in the left arm (arrows) followed a mastectomy and irradiation. A preoperative lymphoscintigram failed to demonstrate a viable lymph node in the left axilla. Reconstructive surgery with free lymph node transplantation was recommended. (B) Donor lymph node-bearing tissue harvested from the right axilla has intact feeding arteries and draining veins making it suitable for free-flap transplantation. It was transplanted from the right to the left axilla using microscopic end-to-end anastomoses (arrows) between donor and recipient arteries and veins. (French method, modified by Becker.) (C) Clinical improvement is evident after surgery (arrows). The patient reported less edema and demonstrated improved range of motion. Lymphoscintigraphy highlighted the newly transplanted lymph nodes in the left axilla (arrows). (Photos courtesy C Becker.)

progression of the disease from stage II to III, often requires a semipermanent commitment to CDT (19).

This need is accentuated when advanced disease dictates a lymphovenous anastomosis at the pop-

liteal level, rather than a standard anastomosis at the inguinal level, which is used in earlier disease stages (24,29). Proximal inguinal lymphatic paralysis would require supplemental CDT to assist in evacuating accumulated proximal edema (29,32).

Evaluation of Bypass Surgery Results

The multidisciplinary care team should evaluate the patient's clinical and laboratory treatment response at least twice annually. Postoperative assessment of treatment response includes infrared optic limb volumetry of the extremity on each visit; lymphoscintigraphy is obtained at 6 months and at each anniversary thereafter. If indicated, an ultrasonographic scan of the limb's veins is added at the end of the follow-up period. When episodes of cellulitis or other sepsis intervene, additional tests may be necessary (32).

Ideally, the results of treatment should be recorded at 1, 2, 3, 6, 12, 18, and 24 months after surgery. It should then be extended from 24 to 48 months, and long-term results should be based on an 8- to 10-year experience.

Clinical Experience

From January 1995 to December 2002, 1065 patients with chronic lymphedema were treated at the Samsung Medical Center in Seoul, South Korea.

Of these, 65 limbs of 54 patients were accepted for surgical treatment because of documented medical treatment failure—disease progression in spite of adequate manual lymph drainage and compression therapy performed for at least a year (11,29,31,32).

Their diagnoses were made with a variety of testing methods—ultrasonography, radionuclide lymphoscintigraphy, magnetic resonance imaging (MRI), and laboratory studies.

Treated limbs were divided into 3 groups:

Excisional surgery group = 22 patients
mean age, 46 years

F = 19, M = 3
primary disease = 5, secondary disease = 17
unilateral disease = 11, bilateral disease = 22

- Lymphovenous anastomotic surgery group = 19
  patients
  ◦ mean age, 49 years
  ◦ F = 18, M = 1
  ◦ primary disease = 4, secondary disease = 15

  Free lymph node transplantation group = 13
  patients

  ◦ mean age, 34 years
  ◦ F= 10, M = 3
  ◦ primary disease = 6, secondary disease = 7

Excisional Surgery Group

Using a modified Homans operation, 6 patients in clinical stage III and the remaining 16 patients in stage IV underwent excisional surgery in a total of 33 lower limbs.

Twenty-eight of the 33 limbs showed an overall improvement at 12 months; of these 28 limbs, 18 were able to retain satisfactory improvement at 24 months only when the patients were compliant with compression therapy. Others in patients with poor compliance failed to maintain improvement. Eight limbs among patients with good compliance to compression therapy maintained good results at 48 months; as with the other groups, poorly compliant patients showed deterioration of their legs, both locally and systemically.

Lymphovenous Anastomotic Surgery Group

All 19 patients in clinical stages I to II selected as candidates for lymphovenous anastomotic surgery met the criteria for progression of disease under adequate treatment. Follow-up assessment was conducted at 24 and 48 months.

Sixteen of the patients, who complied with postoperative CDT, demonstrated clinically satisfactory improvement. The remaining 3 noncompliant patients showed continued deterioration of the limb.

Postoperatively, vigorous CDT was required for all patients as part of the total care management program.

Free Lymph Node Transplantation Group

According to the evaluation criteria, 13 patients, mostly in clinical stages I to II, were selected for surgery. Lymph node-bearing tissue, mainly from the posterior axilla, was transplanted to the inguinal region.

Ten patients compliant with postoperative CDT programs showed clinical evidence of a successful graft at 12 months. The remaining 3 poorly compliant patients failed to prosper.

Summary

When combined with CDT, surgical therapy remains an adjunctive intervention that can help improve the treatment results of selected lymphedema patients. This management approach, however, has lacked popular support because the microsurgical technique demands unerring surgical expertise and a tremendous amount of time and effort. The results remain equivocal as well.

Both excisional and reconstructive surgeries appear to control the progression of lymphedema, at least in early postoperative periods. During follow-up periods ranging between 24 and 48 months, the authors' findings have always shown that long-term results improve when patient compliance with self-initiated CDT is optimal. Free lymph node transplantation-treated limbs also show an improved outcome when accompanied with postoperative CDT, although it is necessary only until transplanted lymph node survival is assured.

To better understand the role of surgical operations in the management of chronic lymphedema, well-constructed trials are warranted. They must consist of well-organized multicenter studies that use similar protocols and incorporate peer-reviewed outcome results. For the future, surgery remains the only possible treatment method capable of providing a cure.

References

1. Theys S, Deltombe TH, Scavée V, et al. Safety of long-term usage of retrograde-intermittent pneumatic compression in lower limb lymphedema. *Lymphology*. 2002;35.
2. Leduc O, Bourgeois P, Leduc A. Manual of lymphatic drainage: scintigraphic demonstration of its efficacy on colloidal protein reabsorption. In: Partsch ed. *Progress in Lymphology IX*. Excerpta Medica. Amsterdam: Elsevier; 1988.
3. Pappas CJ, O'Donnell TF. Long-term results of compression treatment for lymphedema. *J Vasc Surg*. 1992.
4. Hwang JH, Kwon JY, Lee KW, et al. Changes in lymphatic function after complex physical therapy for lymphedema. *Lymphology*. 1999.
5. Foldi E, Foldi M, Weissleder H. Conservative treatment of lymphedema of the limbs. *Angiology*. 1985.
6. Casley-Smith JR, Casley-Smith JR. *Modern Treatment for Lymphoedema*. Adelaide: Lymphoedema Association of Australia; 1994.
7. Hwang JH, Lee KW, Chang DY, et al. Complex physical therapy for lymphedema. *J Korean Acad Rehab Med*. 1998.
8. Hwang JH, Kim TU, Lee KW, et al. Sequential intermittent pneumatic compression therapy in lymphedema. *J Korean Acad Rehab Med*. 1997.
9. Auchincloss H. New operation for elephantiasis. *P R J Publ Health Trop Med*. 1930.
10. Homans J. The treatment of elephantiasis of the legs. *N Engl J Med*. 1936.
11. Kim DI, Huh S, Lee SJ, et al. Excision of subcutaneous tissue and deep muscle fascia for advanced lymphedema. *Lymphology*. 1998.
12. Sistrunk WE. Further experiences with the Kondoleon operation for elephantiasis. *JAMA*. 1918;1:800–805.
13. Kinmonth JB, Patrick J II, Chilvers AS. Comments on operations for lower limb lymphedema. *Lymphology*. 1975.
14. Degni M. New technique of lymphatic-venous anastomosis for the treatment of lymphedema. *J Cardiovasc Surg* (Turin). 1978.
15. Baumeister RGH, Seifert J, Hahn D. Autotransplantation of lymphatic vessels. *Lancet*. 1981.
16. Baumeister RGH, Siuda S. Treatment of lymphedemas by microsurgical lymphatic grafting: what is proved? *Plast Reconst Surg*. 1990.
17. Becker C, Hidden G, Godart S, et al. Free lymphatic transplant. *Eur J Lymphol*. 1991;6:75–80.

18. Becker C, Hidden G, Pecking A. Transplantation of lymph nodes: an alternative method for treatment of lymphedema. *Progr Lymphol*. 1990;6:487–493.
29. Campisi C, Boccardo F, Zilli A, et al. Long-term results after lymphatic-venous anastomoses for the treatment of obstructive lymphedema. *Microsurgery*. 2001.
20. Campisi C, Boccardo F, Zilli A, et al. The use of vein grafts in the treatment of peripheral lymphedemas: long-term results. *Microsurgery*. 2001.
21. Gloviczki P. Review. Principles of surgical treatment of chronic lymphoedema. *Int Angiol*. 1999.
22. Huang GK. Results of microsurgical lymphovenous anastomoses in lymphedema—report of 110 cases. *Langenbecks Arch Surg*. 1989.
23. Krylov VS, Milanov NO, Abalmasov KG, et al. Reconstructive microsurgery in treatment of lymphoedema in extremities. *Int Angiol*. 1985.
24. Krylov VS, Milanov NO, Abalmassov KG. Efficacy of lympho-venous anastomosis. *J Mal Vasc*. 1988.
25. Olszewski WL. The treatment of lymphedema of the extremities with microsurgical lympho-venous anastomoses. *Int Angiol*. 1988.
26. Gloviczki P, Fisher J, Hollier LH, et al. Microsurgical lymphovenous anastomosis for treatment of lymphedema: a critical review. *J Vasc Surg*. 1988.
27. Brorson H. Liposuction gives complete reduction of chronic large arm lymphedema after breast cancer. *Acta Oncol*. 2000.
28. Brorson H. Liposuction in arm lymphedema treatment. *Scand J Surg*. 2003.
29. Lee BB, Kim DI, Hwang JH, et al. Contemporary management of chronic lymphedema—personal experiences. *Lymphology*. 2002.
30. Lee BB. Lymphoedeme post-chirurgical: un terme frappe d'interdiction pour les chirurgiens. *Angeiologie*. 2004.
31. Lee BB. Chronic lymphedema, no more stepchild to modern medicine. *Eur J Lymphology*. 2004.
32. Lee BB. Current issues in management of chronic lymphedema: personal reflection on an experience with 1065 patients. [Commentary.] *Lymphology*. 2005;38.
33. Dellon Al, Hoopes JE. The Charles procedure for primary lymphedema. *Plas Reconstr Surg*. 1977.
34. Lee BB, Bergan JJ. New clinical and laboratory staging to improve management of chronic lymphedema. *Lymphology*. 2005;38.
35. Choi JY, Hwang JH, Park JM, et al. Risk assessment of dermatolymphangioadenitis by lymphoscintig-

raphy in patients with lower extremity lymph-edema. *Korean J Nucl Med.* 1999.

36. Choi JY, Lee KH, Kim SE, et al. Quantitative lympho-scintigraphy in post-mastectomy lymphedema:

correlation with circumferential measurements. *Korean J Nucl Med.* 1997.

37. Slavin S. Liposuction in the consensus document. *Lymphology.* 2004.

7
Chronic Lymphovenous Disease

Lawrence L. Tretbar

Introduction

Although the surgical treatment of lymphedema warrants a thorough discussion, it requires a highly trained and experienced team to obtain successful results, and eligible patients are few.

Lymphovenous disease remains a more prevalent problem than pure lymphedema. However, many physicians experienced in the treatment of early venous diseases are frustrated by the complications of advanced lymphovenous diseases—lipodermatosclerosis, ulceration, cellulitis, lymphovenous edema (phlebolymphedema)—which prevent traditional treatment methods of the venous syndrome.

Healthy Leg Veins

Under normal conditions, venous blood is pumped back to the heart by contractions of the leg muscles, against the pull of gravity. Valves within the veins maintain unidirectional flow and prevent blood from falling backward. But because of our upright stance, there is constant hydrostatic pressure within the leg veins. Fortunately, as blood is pumped away, there is a concomitant fall in pressure. Hydrostatic pressure, altered by exercise, is calculated as ambulatory venous pressure and measured in mmHg. For example, the venous pressure in the foot when an individual stands at rest is about 100 mmHg. When the leg is exercised, the pressure (ambulatory venous pressure) can drop by 20% to 80%. Leg vein health depends on the ability of the valve/muscle system to decrease ambulatory venous pressure during exercise (1,3).

Chronic Venous Insufficiency

As long as venous structures remain healthy and their muscular pumps function properly, fluid entering the interstitial spaces is easily removed by the venules and lymphatics. Should the leakage of fluid from the arteriovenous capillary network increase, lymphatics normally respond by increasing their outflow. If the lymphatics can continue to evacuate the increased fluid load, further damage and edema may be avoided. But if pressure is not attenuated by exercise, the states of chronic venous hypertension and chronic venous insufficiency are created; continued damage to the venous and lymphatic structures is almost inevitable (1–3).

Numerous causes can create valvular incompetence and venous insufficiency, including the inflammatory damage of venous thrombosis, trauma, hereditary factors, or the hormonal effects of pregnancy. Both deep and superficial venous systems may be affected.

Chronic venous insufficiency can develop devastating consequences; high-protein fluid escapes into the interstitial space, and the lymphatics are at risk of damage. In most cases the superficial veins dilate and the valves are unable to prevent reflux—the backward flow of blood. Starling equation is upset by the continued elevation of ambulatory venous pressure and hydrostatic pressure, thereby perpetuating the state of chronic venous hypertension (3–6).

Other causes of venous damage, reflux and swelling include:

Endoluminal Venous Obstruction

- acute deep vein thrombosis—unilateral edema
- acute superficial vein thrombosis—unilateral edema
- combined acute deep and superficial vein thrombosis—marked unilateral edema
- inferior vena caval obliteration, filter, local thrombosis—chronic, marked bilateral edema
- late post-thrombotic syndrome—chronic, may be bilateral edema (see Figure 7-1)

Extraluminal Venous Obstruction

- ruptured medial gastrocnemius muscle head in calf—acute, unilateral edema
- ruptured popliteal synovial (Baker) cyst at knee—acute, unilateral edema

- iliac artery or vein compression—chronic, unilateral edema
- pregnancy—chronic, may be bilateral edema
- chronic distended urinary bladder, stricture, enlarged prostate—chronic, may be bilateral edema
- aortic, iliac, popliteal arterial aneurysm—usually chronic, may be bilateral edema
- malignancy, iliac, intra-abdominal—chronic, usually unilateral
- retroperitoneal fibrosis—chronic, may be bilateral

Muscle Pump Failure/Dependent Leg Syndrome

- spinal cord paralysis or stroke with mobility loss—chronic, bilateral
- confinement to chair—chronic, bilateral
- arthritis with ankle joint fixation—chronic, may be bilateral

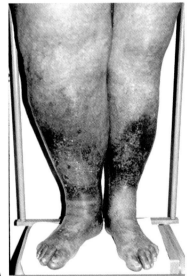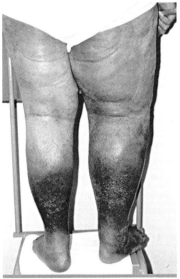

A   B

FIGURE 7-1. (A) This man developed bilateral deep vein thromboses following prolonged bedrest. His legs show all of the complications related to the post-thrombotic syndrome: nonpitting lymphedema of the entire leg, hyperpigmentation, lipodermatosclerosis, and tiny ulcerations in the calves. The feet begin to show the signs of lymphedema—deep flexion creases, puffy feet and toes—but are spared much of the pigmentation because of the compressive effect of tight shoes. (B) Viewed from behind, many of the same features are evident. Note the creases left by his clothing in the upper legs. Swelling obscures Achilles tendons, and pigmentation is circumferential. This patient was not considered a candidate for surgery; his legs were improved with CDT-based treatment and continued compression. (Photos courtesy of LL Tretbar.)

- prolonged travel in car or airplane—acute, usually bilateral
- arterial insufficiency, dependency of leg from pain at rest—chronic, may be unilateral
- prolonged sitting at the computer—acute and chronic, bilateral

Classification of Venous Disease

To classify venous disease, phlebologists developed the Clinical Etiologic Anatomic Pathologic system, known as CEAP. Although this classification system is difficult for many clinicians to use, it is one method of staging venous disease.

Evaluation of Lymphovenous Disease

A thorough history and physical examination are mandatory. Most patients recognize the slowly developing varicose veins from heredity, after trauma, or following pregnancy. Deep vein thrombosis, a potentially serious problem, may resolve completely, or it can cause permanent damage to the leg's venous system. The post-thrombotic syndrome often develops many years after the original deep vein thrombosis and presents with signs and symptoms of chronic lymphedema (3,7–9) (Figure 7-1).

Although many varicose veins appear simple, they too may become totally incompetent and incite progressive damage to the surrounding tissues.

Duplex ultrasonography is the primary method of evaluating the leg for venous disease. A scan of the leg demonstrates both the architecture and function of the venous system. Ultrasound findings are highly reliable, reproducible, noninvasive, and harmless to the tissues. Ultrasonography can also distinguish between superficial and deep vein insufficiency, or a mixture of both (Figure 2-7).

Lymphangioscintigraphy is not useful for evaluating the venous system, but may help distinguish a lymphatic component of the disease process.

Other characteristics help delineate lymphovenous disease from purely lymphatic disease. Cutaneous complications are common to both, but those of chronic venous insufficiency may be more severe. For example, marked hyperpigmentation, not always seen with lymphedema, usually develops in the lower leg, whereas deep skin creases or papillomatosis may not develop (9,10) (Figure 2-6).

Lipodermatosclerosis (thickening and hardening of the skin and subcutaneous tissues), eczematoid dermatitis, ulceration, and loss of joint mobility are frequently distinguishing features of venous disease. These complications are usually accompanied by lymphovenous swelling, and later, pure lymphedema (5,8,11,12) (see Figure 2-5).

Planning a Treatment Program

For the advanced case of chronic venous insufficiency, where secondary complications are present, the initial treatment is similar to that for lymphedema (13–15). A CDT-based treatment program is started to minimize edema, maximize infection control, heal ulcers, and soften lipodermatosclerosis (7,11,13,22).

After these complications have been treated, a re-evaluation of the leg with ultrasonography may help determine later treatment. On occasion the patient may be satisfied with continued compression, or he or she may desire specific treatment for the damaged veins (16,17–20).

The object of treatment is to eliminate venous hypertension by eliminating the reflux of blood. The usual treatment modalities include closure of the offending veins with injections of a sclerosant, as many lymphatic malformations are treated (see chapter 4), and the surgical removal of incompetent veins (21). This alternative may provide a more permanent result.

When both superficial and deep veins are involved, removing the superficial veins (with their overload of blood) can improve deep vein function (3,8,9). Surgical repair of incompetent valves in the deep veins is under investigation but has been only partially successful. It too requires an experienced surgical team to achieve maximum results.

Surgical Techniques

In most cases of advanced venous disease, it is the greater or lesser saphenous vein and their tributaries that are at fault. Complete removal of the

FIGURE 7-2. (A) A flexible stripper is introduced and advanced through the vein that is to be removed. Tiny incisions allow the instrument to remove the veins from beneath the skin with minimal trauma and scarring. (B) A phlebectomy hook draws the side branch varicosities from the subcutaneous tissues. (Photos courtesy of LL Tretbar.)

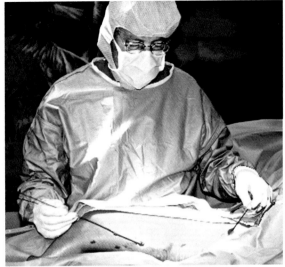

A

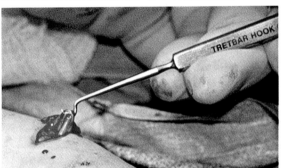

B

damaged veins, or stripping, has been a traditional method of eliminating saphenous veins whose reflux causes venous hypertension. Side branch varicosities are removed with tiny hooks, a technique termed hook phlebectomy (3,9) (Figure 7-2).

Experienced surgeons perform the surgery as an outpatient procedure using local anesthesia, often supplemented with conscious sedation. Continued compression is essential, at least during the healing phase; occasionally, use of compressive garments is discontinued at a later date.

Endoluminal Ablation

Rather than removing the veins, endoluminal ablation closes the incompetent venous conduit that maintains the reflux. This technique obliterates the lumen of the saphenous vein with heat or with injections of a sclerosant (3,17,19) (see chapter 4).

Results of Surgical Treatment

In a 10-month retrospective study of 105 patients who received surgical treatment for lymphovenous disease in 113 legs, one-third had swelling or advanced lymphedema of the limb. Other cutaneous complications were found in 76 limbs.

At the completion of the study, all limbs had improved: hyperpigmentation decreased, lipodermatosclerosis softened, "intractable" ulcers healed, edema and episodes of inflammation and infection were reduced. Only half of the limbs required continued compression, usually in the form of compression garments. The illustrations (Figures 7-3 to 7-5) demonstrate the results of surgical treatment.

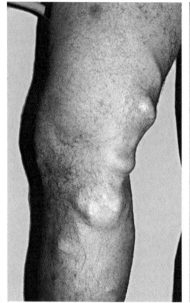 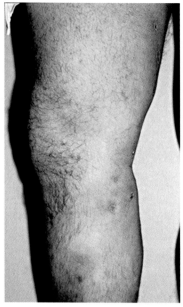

A   B

FIGURE 7-3. (A) Chronic superficial venous disease has dilated the saphenous vein to 3 cm. An otherwise normal muscle pump could not decrease or relieve the resultant venous hypertension. At surgery, the large incompetent saphenous vein was stripped. (B) At 6 weeks following surgery, the bulging veins have disappeared and the multiple incisions were healing well with minimal scarring.

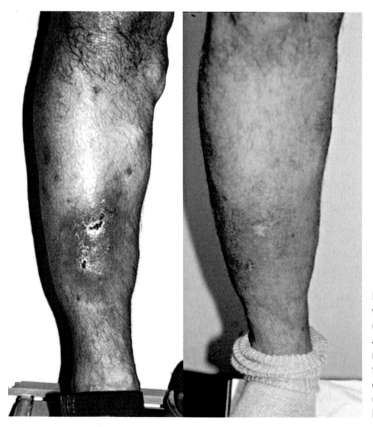

FIGURE 7-4. These images present another view of the leg. In the preoperative photo (left), note the hyperpigmentation, ulcerations, and hair loss. The skin was taut with nonpitting edema. Six years after surgery, the leg has been rehabilitated (right). Most of the pigmentation has lightened, the ulcers have healed, the skin is softened and lost hair has regrown.

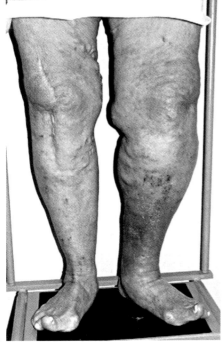

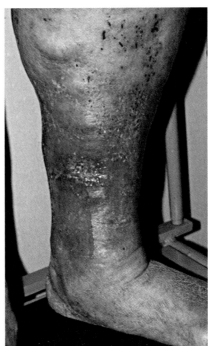

A

B

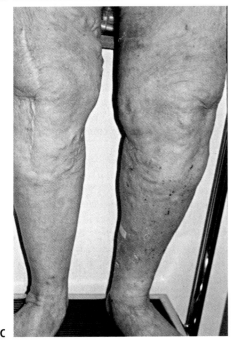

C

FIGURE 7-5. (A) Large varicose veins dominate the medial surface of the left leg. The lower thigh and upper calf contain nonpitting edema. The right leg has had a prosthetic knee replacement. (B) Chronic liposclerosis narrows the lower calf ("bottle leg"), while an intense acute liposclerosis inflames the surface. Clear lymph runs from a shallow ulcer. (C) The complications shown above were first ameliorated with CDT-based medical treatment. Surgery then removed the observable varicose veins and the proximal saphenous trunk. Two years following surgery, the left leg shows neither varicose veins nor swelling. The healed ulcer bed is covered only with tape, and the liposclerotic tissues have softened and lost their inflammation. The foot, however, remains stiff from ankylosed joints. (Photos courtesy LL Tretbar.)

Summary

It is critically important to consider lymphovenous disease during the investigation of the swollen leg. Many patients can receive specific treatment to improve the disease. Although post-thrombotic limbs may not be amenable to direct surgical treatment, those limbs with superficial venous damage may benefit from surgical or medical intervention. Careful sonographic evaluation is essential for the diagnosis (18). Unfortunately, many sonographers only look for deep venous disease and ignore superficial disease. When possible, physicians should perform the testing themselves, or with the vascular technician.

The complications of lymphovenous disease can often be improved with relatively simple treatment (11,14,22). To ignore this possibility is to ignore the best interests of the patient.

References

1. Fegan, WG. *Varicose Veins*. London: Heinemann; 1967.
2. Leu AJ, Leu HJ, Hoffman K, Franzeck UK. Microvascular changes in chronic venous insufficiency—a review. *Cardiovasc Surg*. 1995.
3. Tretbar LL. *Venous Disorders of the Legs*. London: Springer-Verlag; 1999.
4. Bollinger A, Senring G, Franzeck UK. Lymphatic microangiopathy, a complication of severe chronic venous incompetence. *Lymphology*. 1982.
5. Mortimer PS. Implications of the lymphatics system in CVI-associated edema. *Angiology*. 2000.
6. Partsch H, Urbanek A, Wenzel-Hora B. Dermal lymphangiography in chronic venous incompetence. In: Bollinger A, Partsch H, Wolfe JHN, eds. *The Initial Lymphatics*. Stuttgart: Thieme; 1985;178–179.
7. Tiedjen KU, Schultz-Ehrenburg U, Knorz S. Lymphabflussestorengen bei Chronischer Veneninsuffizienz. *Phlebol*. 1992;21:63–71.
8. Browse NI, Burnand KG, Thomas ML. *Diseases of the Veins: Pathology, Diagnosis and Treatment*. London: Arnold; 1988.
9. Bergan JJ, Yao JST. *Venous Disorders*. Philadelphia: Saunders; 1991.
10. Picard J-D. *Venous Circulation*. Lavaur, France: Editions Médicales Pierre Fabre; 1993.
11. Hartmann BR, Drews B, Kayser T. Physical therapy improves venous hemodynamics in cases of primary varicosity: results of a controlled study. *Angiology*. 1997.
12. Browse N, Burnand K, Mortimer P, eds. *Diseases of the Lymphatics*. London: Arnold; 2003.
13. Vodder E. *Die manuelle Lymphdrainage unde medizinishen ihre Anwendungssgebiete*. Erfahrungsheilkunde, 1966;16:7.
14. Piller NB, Swedborg I, Norrefalk JR. Lymphedema rehabilitation program. An application of anatomical, physiological, and pathological knowledge. *Lymphology*. 1992.
15. Casley-Smith JR, Casley-Smith JR. *Modern Treatment for Lymphoedema*. Adelaide: The Lymphoedema Association of Australia; 1994.
16. Blair SD, Wright DDI, Backhouse CM, Riddle E, McCollum CN. Sustained compression and healing of chronic venous ulcers. *BMJ*. 1988.
17. Weissleder H, Schuchhardt C, eds. *Lymphedema: Diagnosis and Therapy*. 2nd ed. Bonn: Kagerer Kommunikation; 1997.
18. Földi M, Földi E. *Methods of Treatment and Control, A Guide for Patients and Therapists*, 5th ed. Newell A, trans. Stuttgart: Gustav Fischer Verlag; 1991; republished by Lymphoedema Association of Victoria, Australia, 1991.
19. Földi M, Kubik S, eds. *Lehrbuch der Lymphologie für Mediziner, Masseure und Physiotherapeuten*, 5th ed. Munich-Jena: Urban & Fisher; 2002.
20. Hutzschenrueter P, Brummer H, Ebberfeld K. Experimental and clinical studies of the mechanisms of effect of manual lymph drainage therapy. *J Lymphology*. 1989.
21. Sigel B, Edelstein A, Savitch L, et al. Types of compression for reducing venous stasis. *Arch Surg*. 1975.
22. Kasseroller RG. *Compendium of Dr. Vodder's Manual Lymph Drainage*. Heidelberg: Haug; 1998.

Index

A

Ablation treatment. *See* Excisional (ablative) treatment
American Society of Lymphology, 44
Angiogenesis, 40, 48
Angio-osteohypertrophy syndrome. *See* Klippel-Trenaunay syndrome
Ankle-brachial pressure index (ABPI), 16
Antibodies, 10
Aplasia, primary lymphedema-related, 31
Arteriovenous malformations, 33
Arthritis, as lymphedema cause, 13
Aselli, Gaspar, 1, 2, 3

B

Bandaging, for lymphedema management, 46, 47, 49–50, 52
Blood circulation, 1
"Bottle leg," 69

C

Cancer, as lymphedema cause, 15–16
Cancer treatment, as lymphedema cause, 13, 14, 24
Cellulitis
  as lymphedema cause, 12, 15, 16, 24
  as lymphovenous disease complication, 64
Children, lymphatic malformation treatment in, 33–34

Classification and staging, of lymphedema, 21–30
staging methods in, 23–29
Clinical Etiologic Anatomic Pathologic System (CEAP), 26, 66
Complete decongestive therapy (CDT), 55
combined with surgical procedures, 55, 56, 57, 58, 59–60, 61
contraindications to, 48–49, 53
development of, 43
for elephantiasis, 44–47
indications for, 53
for truncular lymphedema, 32
as two-phase intervention, 47–52
Comprehensive decongestive physiotherapy (CDP), 43, 44
Comprehensive Decongestive Therapy©, 51–52
Compression garments, 51, 52
Computed tomography
  of extratruncular lymphatic malformations, 33
  of lymphedema, 18, 33

D

Diabetes mellitus, 24
Differential diagnosis, of lymphedema, 12–20
Diffusion, 8–9
Drugs, as edema cause, 15

E

Ectasia, primary lymphedema-related, 31

Edema. *See also* Lymphedema
definition of, 8
differential diagnosis of, 15–20
lymphatic causes of, 12–14
nonpitting, 25
pathophysiology of, 12
pitting, 25
venous causes of, 15
Effleurage, 49
Elephantiasis
  complete decongestion therapy for, 44–47
  lymphostatic, 23
  silica crystal absorption-related, 13, 14
Embolism, pulmonary, 39, 44
Ethanol, as sclerotherapy agent, 33–34
Excisional (ablative) treatment
  endoluminal, for lymphovenous disease, 67
  of extratruncular lymphatic malformations, 33
  of truncular lymphatic malformations, 32
Exercise programs, for lymphedema patients, 50–51

F

Filariasis, 12, 13, 25–26
Fistulae, arteriovenous, 15, 39
Fluid exchange, 8
Free lymph node transplantation, 58–59, 60, 61

G

Gene therapy, for lymphatic
malformations, 40

H

Harvey, William, 1
Hemangioma, 38
cavernous, 38, 39
spontaneous rupture of, 39
Hippocrates, 1
Hunter, John, 1, 3
Hunter, William, 1, 3
Hyperkeratosis, 14, 32
Hyperpigmentation, 46
deep venous thrombosis-related,
17
edema-related, 16, 17
lymphedema-related, 32
lymphovenous disease-related,
67, 68
post-thrombotic syndrome-
related, 65, 66
Hyperplasia, primary
lymphedema-related, 31
Hypertension
chronic venous, 64
venous, 66–67, 68
Hypertrophy, of bone or limbs, 38,
39
Hypoalbuminemia, 15
Hypoplasia, primary lymphedema-
related, 31

I

Immune system/immunity,
9–10
Infection
cutaneous, lymphedema-
associated, 49
as lymphedema cause, 12, 13
during lymphedema treatment,
45, 46
Inflammation, as lymphedema
cause, 13
International Lymphatic Research
Society, 43
International Society of
Lymphology, 44, 47
*Consensus Document on the
Diagnosis and Treatment
of Peripheral Lymphedema*,
23
Interstitial space, fluid within, 8,
12

K

Kaposi-Stemmer sign, 16
Klippel-Trenaunay syndrome, 15

L

Leg veins, healthy, 64
Lipedema, 18–19
Lipodermatosclerosis, 25, 64, 65, 66,
67
Liposclerosis, 69
Liposuction, 56–57
Lymphangiography, 18
Lymphangioma, 12, 33, 40
Klippel-Trenaunay syndrome-
related, 39
Lymphangioma cavernosa, 31, 33
Lymphangioma circumscriptum,
36, 37
Lymphangioma cystic (hygroma),
31, 33–35
Lymphangioma simplex, 33
Lymphangiomatosis, 33, 37, 38
Lymphangiosarcoma, 36
Lymphangioscintigraphy, for
lymphovenous disease
evaluation, 66
Lymphatic Research Foundation,
44
Lymphatic system
embryology of, 4–5
structure and functions of,
1–11
early investigations of, 1–4, 43
lymph capillaries, 5
lymph collectors, 5, 6
lymph ducts, 6–7
lymph nodes, 6–7
lymph precollectors, 5–6
Peyer patches, 6
prelymphatic tissue channels,
5
Lymph ducts, structure and
functions of, 6–7
Lymphedema
bilateral, chronic stage III, 44–47
chronic, 31
congenital, 22–23
diagnostic tests for, 16, 18
filiarial, 44
hereditary
type II (Meige disease), 12
type I (Milroy disease), 12, 13
primary, 12, 31–32
classification of, 21–22

as lymphangiosarcoma cause,
36
secondary, 12–14, 31
classification of, 22–23
Lymphedema praecox, 12, 22
Lymphedema tarda, 12, 22
Lymph nodes, structure and
functions of, 6–7
Lymphogranuloma venereum, 12
Lymphography, of manual lymph
drainage, 48
Lymphology, 23
Lymphoscintigraphy
of cancer treatment-related
lymphedema, 14
of extratruncular lymphatic
malformations, 33
for lymphedema diagnosis, 16,
18
for lymphedema staging, 26
of manual lymph drainage, 48
preoperative, 56, 58, 59, 60, 61
of primary lymphedema, 31,
32
Lymphovenous disease. *See also*
Venous insufficiency,
chronic
causes of, 64, 65–66
chronic, 64–70
classification of, 66
complications of, 64
evaluation of, 16, 17, 66
surgical treatment of, 66–69

M

Magnetic resonance imaging
of extratruncular lymphatic
malformations, 33
of lipedema, 18
of lymphedema, 18, 32–33
Malformations, lymphatic, 12,
31–42
congenital vascular
malformations associated
with, 38–39
extratruncular forms of, 31,
33–35
gene therapy for, 40
truncular forms of, 31–32, 39
Manual lymph drainage, 46,
48–49
Mascagni, Paulo, 1, 4
Medical management, of
lymphedema, 45–54

historical review of, 45–46
successful, 46–47
as two-phase intervention,
47–52
Meige disease, 12
Microcirculation, 5
Milroy disease, 12, 13
Muscle pump failure/dependent
leg syndrome, 65–66

N
National Lymphedema Network,
44
Nutritional counseling, 51

O
Obesity
as lipedema cause, 19
as lymphedema cause, 24, 51
OK-432, as sclerotherapy agent,
33–34
Osmosis, 9

P
Palliative care, 52
Panniculitis, sclerosing, 25
Papilloma, 46
Peyer patches, 6
Phlebectomy, hook, 67
Phlebolymphedema, 64
Pneumatic pumps, 51
Podoconiosis, 13, 14
Port-wine stain, 38, 39
Post-thrombotic syndrome, 65, 66
Psychosocial interventions, with
lymphedema patients, 52

Q
Quality of life, assessment of,
27–28

R
Reconstructive surgery, lymphatic,
55, 57–58, 59

S
Sclerotherapy, 34–35, 38, 67
Scrofula, 12
Self-management, of lymphedema,
44, 47–48, 52
Skin care, in lymphedema patients,
49
Starling equation, 8
Stewart-Trevers sarcoma. *See*
Lymphangioma
Surgery, as lymphedema cause, 13
Surgical management
of lymphedema, 55–63
clinical outcomes in, 60–61
combined with complete
decongestive therapy
(CDT), 55, 56, 57, 58, 60, 61
excisional/ablation surgery,
55–57, 61, 67
free lymph node
transplantation, 58–59, 60,
61
liposuction, 56–57
lymphatic reconstructive
surgery, 55, 57–58, 59
lymphovenous anastomotic
surgery, 55, 57–58, 59, 61
postoperative management in,
59–60
vein grafting, 59
of lymphovenous disease, 66–69

T
Thrombosis
deep venous, 17, 65
as venous insufficiency cause, 64

Trauma
as lipedema cause, 19
as lymphedema cause, 13, 14,
15
as venous insufficiency cause,
64
Tuberculosis, of the lymph nodes,
12

U
Ulcers
deep venous thrombosis-related,
17
dressings for, 46, 49
elephantiasis-related, 45,
46
infection-related, 17
lymphovenous disease-related,
16, 64, 65, 66, 67, 68,
69
Ultrasonography, duplex,
17
for lymphovenous disease
evaluation, 66, 70

V
Varicose veins, 22, 38, 45, 66, 67,
69
Vascular malformations,
congenital, 38–39
Vasculogenesis therapy, 40
Vein grafting, as lymphedema
treatment, 59
Venous insufficiency, chronic
as lipedema cause, 19
as lymphedema cause, 14, 15, 16,
24, 64–70

W
Wound care, 46, 49